AF553776

Standardization and Pharmacological Evaluation of Plants

Vimal Kumar Singh

A.P.H. PUBLISHING CORPORATION
4435–36/7, ANSARI ROAD, DARYA GANJ,
NEW DELHI-110002

Published by
S.B. Nangia
A.P.H. Publishing Corporation
4435–36/7, Ansari Road, Darya Ganj,
New Delhi-110002
Phone: 011–23274050
e-mail: aphbooks@gmail.com

2024

Typeset by
Ideal Publishing Solutions
C-90, J.D. Cambridge School,
West Vinod Nagar, Delhi-110092

Printed at
BALAJI OFFSET
Navin Shahdara, Delhi-110032

Dedicated

to

My Beloved Parents

PREFACE

The author feel great pleasure in presenting the book "STANDARDIZATION AND PHARMACOLOGICAL EVALUATION OF PLANTS", with increasing the interest in the field of herbal medicines, cosmetics, Ayurvedic dosage forms and research in the field of herbal formulations. This book is a very important for students of branch pharmaceutical education and it gives stepwise information required during practical performing. It provides knowledge of different techniques or different steps involve in the standardization of plants. It provides pharmacological activities and animal handling.

- This book is useful for the students of B.Pharm, M.Pharm and Pharm-D.
- The author highly appreciate the work of publishing staff of APH Publishing Corporation, New Delhi.
- Your cooperation in the form of suggestions and comments are most welcome.

ACKNOWLEDGEMENT

I take this golden opportunity to express my gratitude and sincere thanks towards my supervisor Prof.P.K.Sharma, (Director & Head), Institute of Pharmacy, BundelKhand University, Jhansi, for his excellent guidance and dedicated efforts, and constant encouragement of interest and providing excellent infrastructure facilities for my research work for the successful comletion of this thesis work. Without his well-directed instructions, proper guidance, good advice and moral support, this thesis would not have taken a fruitful shape.

I am very much thankful to my co-guide Dr.Vidhu Aeri, Sr. Lecturer, Deptt. Of Pharmacognosy & Photochemistry, his meticulous guidance, consistent encouragement, patience listening and perspective criticism in shaping this dissertation. All the valuable advice given by his will remain treasure.

I expressly wish to thank Mrs. Raj Kumari, Ph.D. Scholer, Deptt. Of Pharmacy, Jamia Hamdard University, New Delhi, who had read, criticized and corrected mistakes with special interest and give excellent guidance.

I am grateful to Dr. Arvind Bhardwaj, Botanist, Natural drugs & Botanicals, Ghaziabad (U.P.), for identified drug sample for my research work.

I am thankful to Dr. R.S. Chauhan, Joint Director, Dr.A.G. Telang, Senior Scientist, Mr. Harish Chandra, Technical officer & Mr. Sudhir, Technical officer, Deptt. Of CADRAD, I.V.R.I., Izatnagar (U.P.) for support during my dissertation work.

I am thankful to Dr. Mahesh Gupta, Dr. Sunil k. Prajapati, Dr. Raghurveer Irchiaya, Dr.S.K.Jain. Mr.A.K.Jain, Mr.S.Palani & Mrs. Nisha Joseph Plani, for their co-operation in all respects.

I would like to thanks to Dr. Rajdeep, Reader, Deptt. Of Botany, Budelkhand University, Jhansi, for important Guidance in completion of microscopic studies.

I would like thanks to all Non-teaching staff specially Vivek sir, Nayak sir, Shukla sir, Naresh sir, & Birju for Support During my dissertation work.

I also thanks to all my friends specially for Pushpendra, Nandlal, Ritesh, Nagesh, Suneel, P.yadav, Santoshi, Mansing, Ashok gupta, Mahindra Rana for their kind support time to time.

I am also grateful to my dear Juniors for thair support Hemant, Neeraj, Pradeep, Vineet, & Hassam Uddin Khan.

I am also express my regards to library of INSDOC, New Delhi, Deptt. Library & central library of Jamia Hamdard University, IVRI library, Bareilly, and Deptt. Library of Institute of Pharmacy, Bundelkhand University, Jhansi, for assistance in the survey and Procurement of literature.

Finally, this work has been a reality due to the love and encouragement to my beloved Parents, Brothers and Sisters.

Vimal Kumar Singh

CONTENTS

ABOUT THE AUTHOR

Mr. Vimal Kumar Singh is working as an Assistant Professor, Pharmacognosy, Department of Pharmacy, M.J.P. Rohilkhand University, Bareilly, Uttar Pradesh. He has more than 5 years of teaching and research experience. His areas of interest in different parameters of standardization technique, different pharmacological activities and design many experiments at B.Pharm level. He has guided a number of B.Pharm students and published several research papers in National and International Journals. He is a member of Board of Studies, Department of Pharmacy, M.J.P. Rohilkhand University, Bareilly, Uttar Pradesh.

Chapter-1

INTRODUCTION

"Opportunities for development of modern phytomedicines based on Pharmacognosist"

In our country we have well accepted classical system of treatments like Ayurveda, Unani and Siddha. These are getting dominant over each other at different ages due to many socio-economic and potential reasons. All these utilize potentials of natural products or materials of natural origin for curing various disorders and health hazards.

Various researches are going even today based on ancient system of treatment from natural substances used by Charaka, Shushrutha's period. As science advances, people are interested in utilizing only the potential components. So scientists started isolation, identification and purification of chemical and natural moiety, which is mainly responsible for pharmacological or therapeutic action.(Sukhdev., 1997)

It is needless to mention why natural products are preferred over synthetic or the advantages of natural over synthetic ones. They are relatively more safer with minimum side effects. At present research is going on to the maximum extent for utilization of natural products for their best applications. Therefore the phytochemical research mainly deals with utilization of natural origin potentials of plant source for desired pharmacology. It may be for curing or improving various abnormalities of normal health. Even research is going on utilization of natural medicines for HIV causing AIDS, which is a challenge at present millennium in the field of medicine.(Sukhdev. et. al., 1997. Puspangadan. et. al., 1995)

The Phytochemical research is discussed as a chain of events beginning and ending with traditional medicine. Some of the links in this are highlighted in this chain. (puspangadan., et. al, 1995)

- Ethno botanical investigation.
- Selection and collection of the plant material.
- Extraction.
- Bio-assays.
- Isolation of active constituents.
- Structure elucidation.
- Pharmacological investigation.
- Toxicological investigation.
- Chemo taxonomy.
- Plant cultivation.
- Standardization.

There are many systems working through out the world, which includes Chinese traditional, Ayurveda, Unani etc. However, in India "The Local Health Tradition" is the team exclusively dealing with "Stream of Indian Folk Medicine". About 6000 to 7000 plants have been utilized by this committee.

Classically higher plants have played a dominant role in the introduction of new therapeutic agents. On a global basis at least 130 drugs of all single chemical entities extracted from higher plants are modified further synthetically are currently used.

Japanese pharmacopoeia (1986) contains 123 plants both crude and pure active principles of which only 29 are used in western medicine. Plant derived drugs constitute important monograph in the German and Russian pharmacopoeia. Even now almost 75-80% of the world population depends on crude plant drugs preparations to tackle their health problems, though this may be mostly because of economic reasons.

In the period 1950-70 there was introduction of approximately 100 basic new drugs in USA market. This list contained not more than 4 herbal drugs- Reserpine, Recinnamide, Vinblustine and Vincristine derived from higher plants. Again during next (1971-90) over 600 new chemical entities (NCE's) were launched worldwide. Of which many are of natural origin like Temposides etoposide Ñ tetrahydrocannabind, Nabilone, Guggulsterone. At present (1991-96) introduction of 200 NCE's globally of which many 40-60 were of natural (higher plant constituents) Paclitaxel, Iriotecan, Topotecan cromshin, Phylanethin.

Natural Cancer Institute (USA) beginning in 1959 screened over 180,00 plants extracts cover 3500 plant genera during a 20-25 year period.

Central Drug Research Institute (Lucknow, India) screened approximately 2500 plants for wide range pharmacological activities of those b-lactin, quinolone, anti-bacterials, b-blockers, Inhibitors of angiotensin converting enzyme (ACE) histamine and H_2- receptor antagonists. (Ethnobotany., 4th June, 2005)

In spite of so much potential and scope of future development of plant drugs we have not achieved benefit of even 2% of the total flora provide by nature. The major pitfalls in the plant drug research include lack of standardization, confusion in nomenclature, controversial botanical identification, danger of extinction of some plants being extensively over exploited, lack of proper dosage formulations, or frustrating experiences of searching for single active principle. Therefore future of plant drugs depends upon the maintenance of quality control, standardization, therapeutic credibility, proper research funding and our sincere commitment to research on plant drugs.

STANDARDIZATION

Herbs have formed an integral part of our lives since times immemorial. Along with flood and shelter they also provided an immense contribution in maintaining human health. Traditional use of herbal medicine, practiced for more than a thousand years, is the very basis and integral part of various cultures. Almost 65-80% of the world's population still relies on herbal medicines.

The problem of standardization of plant arises from the complex composition of drugs which are sude in the form of crude drugs or plant extracts where major constituents are present. So, there is need for the standardization of traditional drugs for obtaining consistent composition and to ensure predetermined potency of the drug. Therefore, it is standardized on the basis of their chemical constituents. Active principles are preferred for this purpose, in case of the plants where the active principle have not been isolated, other characterizing compounds can be selected as a marker compounds for standardization. Therefore standardization of drugs based on the chemical constituents are most important.

Standardization of plant drug can be done through following parameters i.e.

- Authentication
- Foreign matter
- Organic evaluation
- Microscopical examination
- Moisture content
- Rf values
- Volatile matter
- Ash value
- Extractive values
- Swelling index
- Foaming index
- Crude fibre
- Bitterness value
- Hemolytic activity
- Chromatographic profile & marker component
- Pesticides residues
- Heavy metals
- Microbial contamination
- Total solids
- Tannins
- Radioactive contamination

ANTI-INFLAMMATORY ACTIVITY

Anti-inflammatory drugs are used in various inflammatory disorders such as rheumatoid arthritis, rheumatic fever etc. But due to the side effects their use have taken asset back. Therefore, the research is still continuing for development of better therapeutic agents with least side effect (Turner, 1965).

Rheumatoid disease are characterized by chronic inflammation, it is common practice to test compounds for anti-inflammatory activity then hopefully predict that active once should be useful as anti-rheumatic drugs. Clinically anti-inflammatory drugs are judged by their effect on pain, stiffness or swelling of the affected part the action on swelling being most objectively observable, therefore most important.

Following in vivo experimental models are used for evolution of anti-inflammatory activity.

- Acutre model : Carageenan – induced rat paw oedema(Winter *et al,* 1962)
- Sub-acute model : Formalin – induce arthritis in rats(Selye, 1949)
- Chronic model:Cotton pellet granulomatest in rats, *(D'Arcy et al.* 1960)

ANTI BACTERIAL ACTIVITY

Human kind has been subjected to infections by micro-organisms since before the dawn of recorded history. One presumed that mankind has been searching for suitable therapy for nearly as long.

This was a desperately difficulty enterprise given the acute nature of most infections and the nearly total lack of understanding of their origins, which was prevalent until the last century.

The potential of microorganism is tremendous as for as their beneficial effects are concerned. Several microorganism however, are detrimental and perhaps outweigh the beneficial effects with respect to health and human kind. The increased resistant of microorganism to various drugs is also a cause of alarm. Several researches had been carried out in search of such drugs will be susceptible to different microorganism and also be active against a broad spectrum of microbes.

Those which act against wide range are called broad spectrum antibiotics and those with short range are; known as narrow spectrum antibiotics.

There may be wide variations in the susceptibility of different strains of the same bacterial species to antimicrobial agents. Essential to the choice of drug is information about the pattern of sensitivity of the infecting micro-organisms.

Several tests are now available for determination of bacterial sensitivity to anti-microbial agents. The inhibition of microbial growth under standardized conditions may be utilized for demonstrating the therapeutic efficacy of test compounds. Any change in the anti-microbial molecule, which may not be detected by chemical methods, will be revealed by a reduction in the anti-microbial activity & hence microbiological assays are very useful for resolving doubts regarding possible change in potency of test compound, microbiological assay is based upon a comparison of the inhibition of growth of bacteria by measured concentration of a standard preparation of the antibiotic having a known activity two general methods are generally applied the cylinder plate (or cup plate)methods and the turbidimetric (or tube assay) method. (Michael.J.P., et. al., 2000)

Indian Materia media provides lots of information on the folklore practices and important natural products. Materia media includes about 2000 drugs of natural origin almost all of which are derived from different traditional system and folklore practice. More than 1500 remedial treatments with Indian medicinal flora have been reported by Sushrathasamhith, Charaka Samhita and Veghatta Sanskrit literature written by them contains information about Morphological features of many plants drugs, their geographical distribution and condition of growth is best in season for their maximum potency.

Herbal medicine are of great importance to the health of the individual and communities, but their quality assurance needs to be developed.

In many developed countries there has also been a growing interest in herbal medicine. In India, the ayurvedic system of medicine developed an extensive use of medicines from plants dating from atleast 1000 B.C. (Mukherjee. P.K., 2000)

The plant ***Gloriosa superba Linn.*** Belonging from Liliaceae family is an important medicinal plant. Both seeds and tubers of this plant are used in medicine. Seeds are the rich source of colchicine which are used in preparation of drugs against gout and rheumatism in modern medicine for induction of polyploidy and in botanical researches. Its tubers are used as tonic, antiperiodic, anthelmentic, antiinflammatory and also against snake bite in Indian system of medicine since time immemorial. It is used traditionally in treatment of abortifacient, leprosy, cancer, piles. (Henry.G.G.,1999)

Chapter-2

REVIEW OF LITERATURE

PLANT PROFILE

Gloriosa superba Linn., belonging to the Liliaceae family is an important medicinal plant. Both seeds and tubers of this plant are used in medicine. Seeds are the rich source of colchicines, which is used in the preparation of drugs against gout and rheumatism in modern medicine for induction of polyploidy and in botanical researches. (Farooqi.A.A, et al, 1999)

Several allied species of G. Superba Linn., are the G. simplex Linn., G. grandiflora, G. lutea, G. Plantii, G. leopoldii, G. longifolia, G. rothschildiana, G. virescens and G. sudanica are distributed mainly in Africa. (Farooqi.A.A, et al, 1993)

The plant is grown for its colorful cut flowers and tubers, which yield colchicines and other alkaloids. It is a diploid (2n=22) and fails to successfully cross with other allied species and cultivars, including the native species, G. rothschildiana, an octoploid (2n=88).(Wealth of India, 2002; Vijaya Valli. B., et.al., 1992)

BIOLOGICAL SOURCE

Bot.Name	-	*Gloriosa superba Linn.*
Kingdom	-	Plantae
Division	-	Angiospermae
Class	-	Monocotyledoneae
Order	-	Liliiflorae
Family	-	Liliaceae
Genus	-	Gloriosa
Species	-	*Superba. D.C* (Mukherjee P.K., 2000)

VERNACULAR NAMES

Hindi	-	Kalihari,Languli,Karihari,Kariari
Eng.	-	Superb lily
Beng.	-	Ulat chandal
Sans.	-	Langalika,agnishikha,Kalikari,Garbha-gatini, sukra Pushpika
Tam.	-	Katijan
Tel.	-	Agui-shekka
Malyal.	-	Mavdoni
Duk.	-	Nat-ka-bachanag
Burm.	-	Sunnu-dav
Can.	-	Radagari
Guz.	-	Khadya-naga
Mar.	-	Nagakaria,nagamodia
Kon.	-	Vaganankta

(Antony.R.T., 1996; kapoor.L.D.,)

GEOGRAPHICAL DISTRIBUTION

In India- Throughout tropical India, ascending upto 7000ft. on the hills. This elegant climbing ornamental plant is common in Bengal and low Jungles throughout India. The drug is obtained on a large scale from Tamilnadu, in the tropical forest of Bengal, Karnataka, Bundelkhand and Assam Valleys. (Wealth of India., 2002)

In World- It is well adapted to different soil & climatic variations also formed in Sri Lanka, Burma, Africa common in Mysore State. (Kapoor.L.D.; Kokate.C.K.,et.al., 2001)

CULTIVATION

The plant is a perennial vine crop and remains in the field for several years. It is well adapted to different soil types and climatic variations from arid Bundelkhand to Humid Assam Valley. Small plantations in Karnataka and Tamilnadu. Both the states, having equitable climate, provide favorable conditions to the vines to flower early and for a longer period to make it a viable plantations crop.

It grows luxuriantly in warm weather with a rainfall of 200 cm distribute evenly throughout the year. High temperature and High relative humidity in early period result in vigorous growth.

The rise in temperature from 15^{0}C to 20^{0}C during the day and 10^{0}C to 15^{0}C at night is ideal for copious flowering and seed set.

Medium sandy loam soil having PH of 6-7 is better suited for its cultivation.

The plants can be raised both from seeds and tubers. Treatment of the seeds with Thiourea (0.3-0.4%) gives the maximum germination (67.5%) and maximum rate of germination. The seed propagate plants take 3-4 years to bloom. Hence propagation through tubers is preferable. The land should be ploughed and harrowed to a fine tilth. The leveled field is then divided into small plots, providing slope for drainage. About 15-20 tonnes/ha of farmvard manure or compost is mixed in the soil.

(Farooqi.A.A.,et.al., 1993)

The tuber are brittle, hence their ends must be protected from damage. The apical pieces (50-60g) of tuber should be cut and treated with 0.08% fungicide Emisan-6 for 3 minutes and plants at 6 cm depth in furrows 45-60 cm apart. The row-to-row distance should be maintained at 30-45 cm. The vigour of the growing vines depends upon the tuber weight closer spacing helps cross-fertilization leading to improved fruit set.

A dose of 40kg N, 50kg P_2O_5 and 75 kg K_2O per hectare should be applied at the time of planting and 80 kg N as top dressing 8 weeks after planting. (Kumaraswamy.B.K.,et.al.,1994) The 3 irrigation in a month requires. The crop should not be irrigated after flowering because high soil moisture may cause rotting of the tubers. Chemical weed control is possible only under wide spacing.

If planted in June, the plants start flowering 55 days after planting and the pods mature in about 110 days after flowering.

The pods are picked manually and dried in shade for 7-10 days. The seeds are also dried in shade for a week and then sun dried for another week.

One hectare plantation yields about 150kg seeds in the first year and 250-300kg seeds from the second year on wards. The seeds should be packed in moisture proof containers/bags and stored in a cool, dry place. (Saravanan.S.,et.al., 2003; Wealth of India, 2002)

DESCRIPTION

It is a tall herbaceous climber. The viny stems bear simple stalkless, linear lanceolate leaves with cirrosed tips spirally twisted in the upper part to serve as tendrils.(Farooqi.A.A., et.al.,1993) Leaves terminating in tendril-like, long, curling tips. Leaves alternate, rarely opposite or in whorls, egg-shaped-lanceolate, stalkless, about 5-15 X 2-4cm, base heart shaped, apex produced into a coiled tendril, margin entire hairless, papery; lateral news parallel.

The flowers are in shades of crimson, red, pink, maroon and purple-crisped tepals. The flower bud is green, yellow on opening, changing soon to orange-red and turning to dark pink on red when in full bloom by late autumn. (Farooqi. A.A.,et.al., 1993)

Flowers bisexual, axillary, solitary or somewhat sub-corymobose at the ends of branches, 8-10cm across. Floral stalk 6-14cm long with reflexled apex. Perianth lobes 6, oblong-lanceolate, about 6X1cm, with crisply wavy margins, greenish at first, then yellow, passing through arrange a scarlet to crimson colour. Capsules ellipsoid-oblong, 3-5 X 1-2.5cm, splitting by 3-values.(Duke.J.A.,1929; Swarmapriya.R.,et. al., 1995)

Tubers solid, fleshy, cylindric, white, very long. The rhizomes are cylindrical on slightly flattened with bitter taste fibres are present. 15-25 X 2.5-4 cm, pointed at both ends, 'V' or 'L' shaped Branchlets hairless, weak, and vascular bundles are collateral with slight extensions on both sides of xylem. Starch grains show concentric striations and measure 11 to 38micron in diameter. Seeds numerous, globose, dorsally compressed, with warty projections, straw-colored.

CHEMICAL COMPOSITION

- **LEAVES-** leaves contain 3-desmethylcolchicine $C_{21}H_{23}NO_6$, colchicine $C_{22}H_{25}NO_6$, and chelidonic acid, Di methyl colchicines, N-Formyl deacetyl colchicines, Lumi colchicines. (Indian Pharmacopoeia 1996)
- **FLOWERS-** flowers contain beta-lumicolchicine,$C_{22}H_{25}NO_6$, N-formyldesacetyl-colchicine,$C_{21}H_{23}NO_6$, and 3- desmethyl colchicines.
- **TUBERS-** Tubers contain 0.36% colchicines, N-formyldesacetyl colchicines, 2- desmethyl colchicines, beta-lumicolochicine,gloriosine $C_{33}H_{38}N_2O_9$ or $C_{15}H_{17}NO_4$,gloriosol,$C_{33}H_{56}O_6$ which may represent a mixture of sitostorol and stigmosterol resinous substances 3-demethyl colchicines, 1,2-didemethyl colchicines, 2,3-didemethyl

colchicine,N-for-myl-N-deacetyl colchicines and colchicocide,traces of choline, benzoic acid, salicylic acid, 6-methyl oxysalicylic acid,fatty acids, glucose, starch, γ-rsorcylic acid, monomethyl ether etc.

- **SEEDS**- Seeds contain following alcolides gloriosine, colchicine, superbine.In the world market,they are considered a rich source of colchicines and gloriosine.(Wealth of India,P.180, 2002; Duke.J.A.,1929)

CHEMICAL STRUCTURES

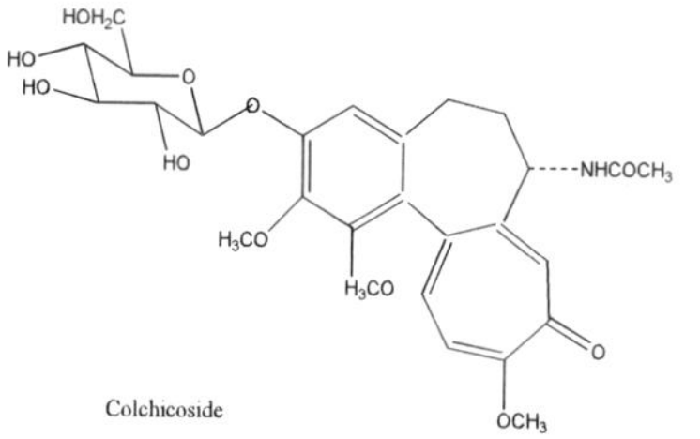

Colchicoside

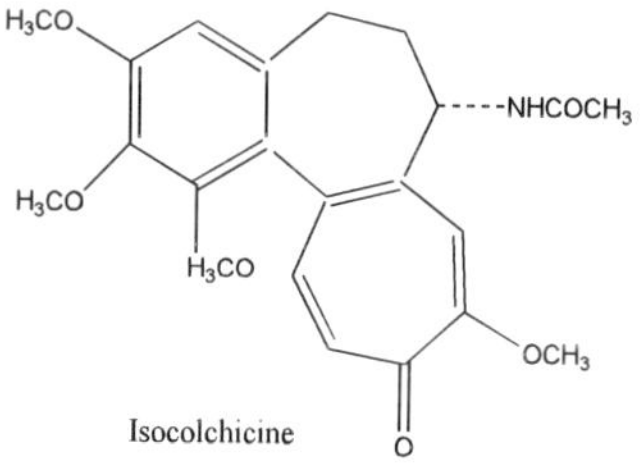

Isocolchicine

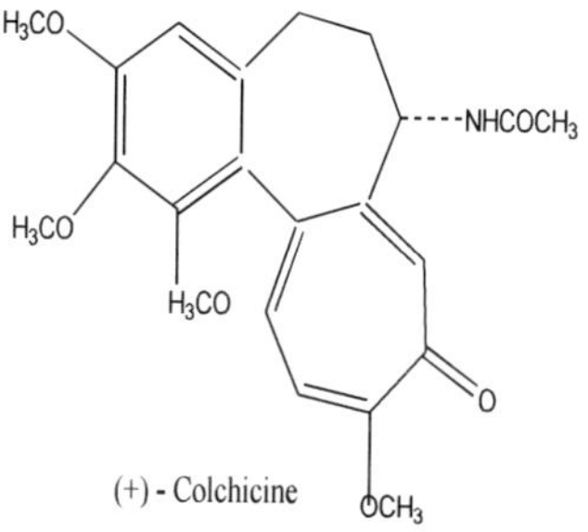

(+) - Colchicine

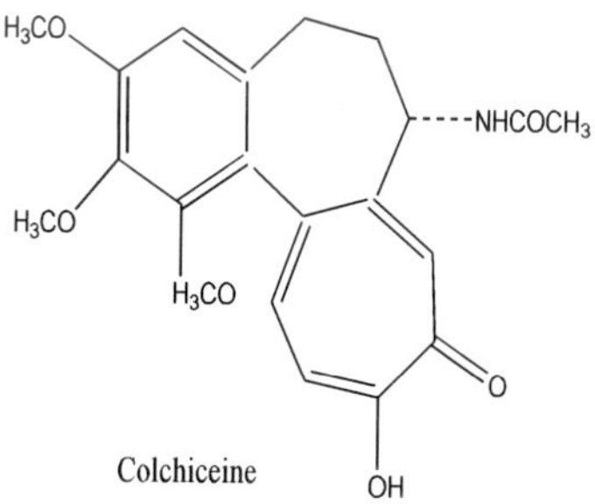

Colchiceine

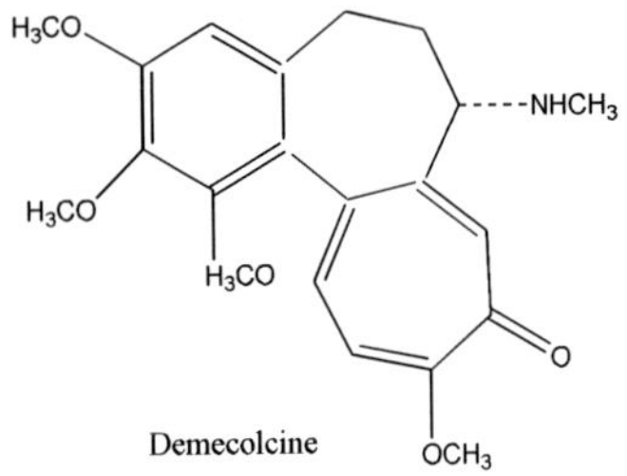

Demecolcine

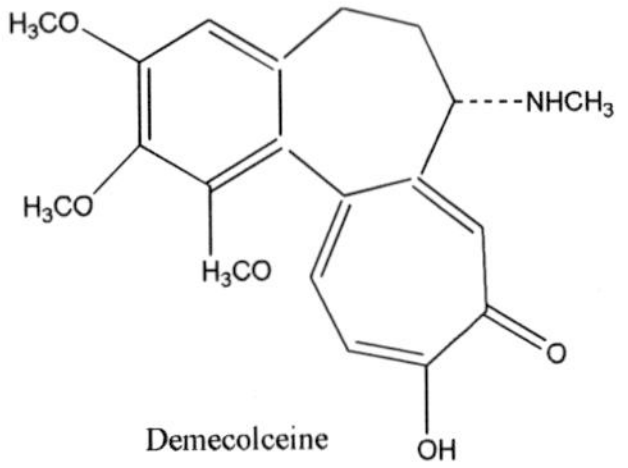

Demecolceine

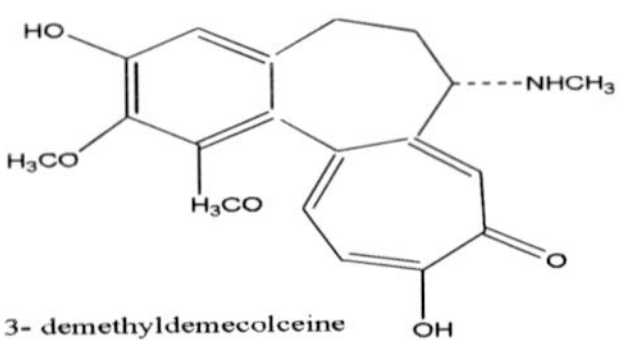

3- demethyldemecolceine

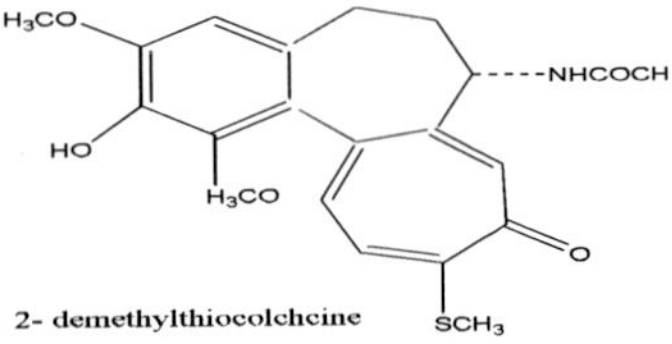

2- demethylthiocolchcine

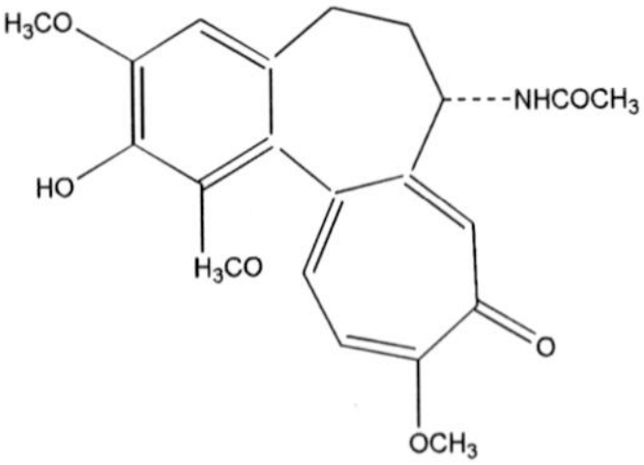

2- demethylcolchicine

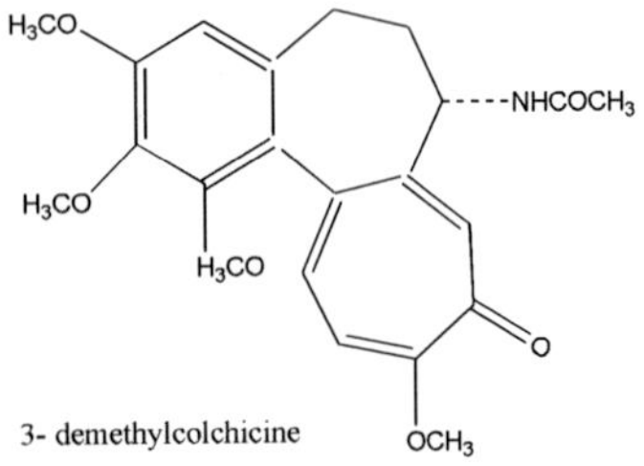

3- demethylcolchicine

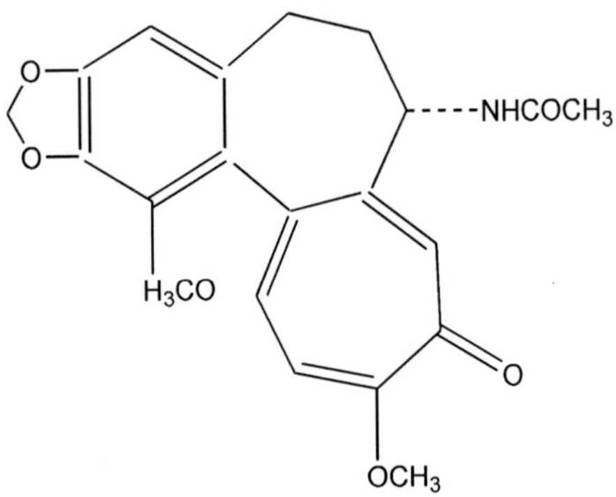

Cornigerine

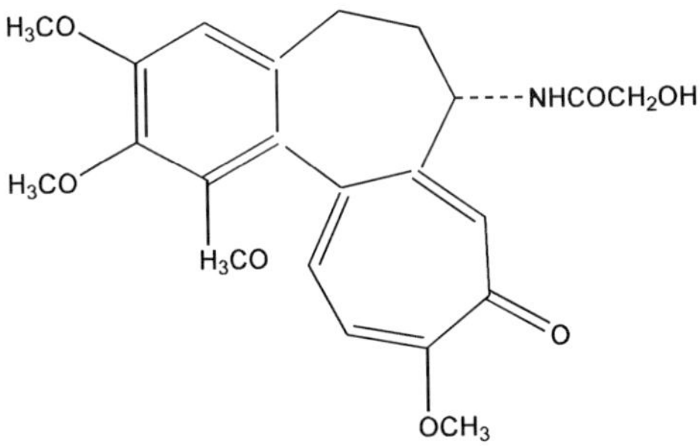

Colchifoline

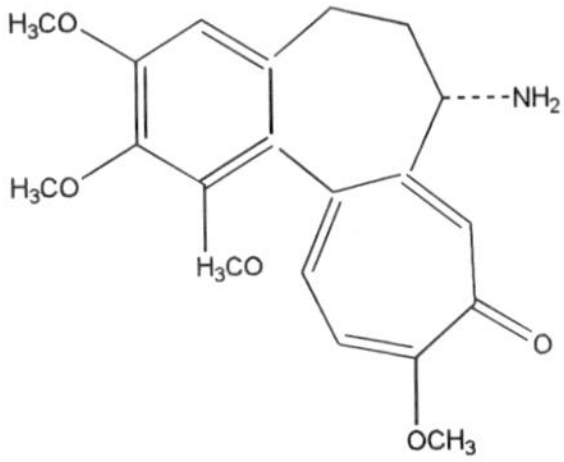

N-deacetylcolchicine

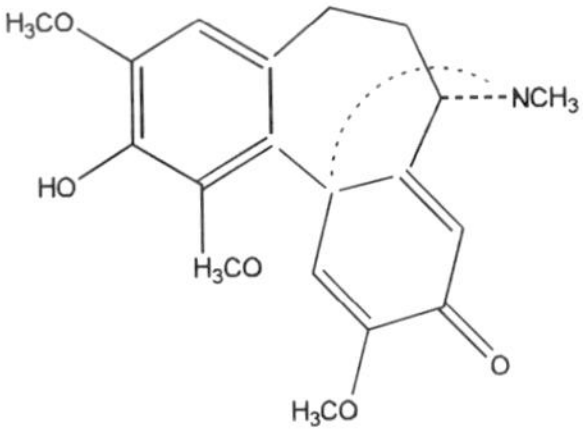

androcymline

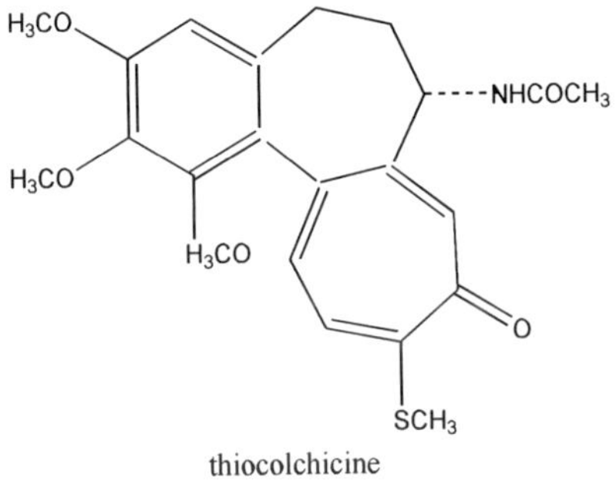

thiocolchicine

(Poulev. A.,et. al., 1994;Sharma.A.K.,et.al.,1986)

USES OF DIFFERENT PARTS

The seeds and tubers are used for medicinal purposes. The tuberous roots are useful in curing inflammation, ulcers, scrofula, bleeding plies, white discharge, skin diseases, leprosy, indigestion, helmenthiasis, snake bites, baldness, intermittent fever and debility. It is used internally as antidote for snake poison. It is considered useful in promoting labour and expulsion of the placenta, gonorrhoea, abortifacient, expel intestinal worms, cancer, colic, malaria, syphilis, tumors, ulcers.(Wealth of India, P.180, 2002)

Seeds are used for rheumatic pain and as a muscle relaxant. If taken in large doses, it is highly poisonous, it causes vomiting, purging, stomachache and burning sensation. (Duke.J.A.,1929)

PHARMACOLOGICAL INVESTIGATION

- Nidiry. E.S.I., et. al., (1996), Reported the Invitro Nematicidal activity of *Gloriosa superba Linn.* Seeds Extract against Meloidogyne incognita(nematode).
- Saily. A., et. al., (1994), Reported the mineral elements of *Gloriosa superba Linn.* Used for the treatment of Asthma, Syphilis, Diarrhoea, Skin diseases and Rheumatism.
- Chandravadana. M.V., et. al., (1999), Reported the Nematicidal activity of *Gloriosa superba Linn.* Plant Extract.
- Subashini. R., et. al., (2000), Reported the Antimicrobial activity of leaf Extraction of *Gloriosa superba Linn.*
- Gupta. K.R., et. al., (2003), Reported the Hepatoprotective activityof *Gloriosa superba Linn.*.

PHYTOCHEMICAL INVESTIGATION

- Arambewela. L.S.R., et. al., (1991), Reported the highest content of total Alkaloids(0.6-0.9%) and Colchicine(0.15-0.25%) are found in the seeds.
- Chaudhuri. P.K., et. al., (1993), Reported a new alkaloid 1,2-Didemethyl colchicines from the *Gloriosa superba Linn.*.
- Chaudhuri. P.K., et. al., (1993), Reported the substitute of colchicines from the plant Colchicum autumnale Linn..
- Poulev. A., et. al., (1994), Reported the Immunoassays for the quantitative determination of Colchicine.
- De-EKnamkul. W., et. al., (1996/97), Reported the Percentage of Colchicine in the different plant parts of *Gloriosa superba Linn.*
- Amal. J.A., et. al., (1998),Reported the Preparation of drug from *Gloriosa superba Linn.* Tubers to cure Leprosy& cancer.

- Chaudhurri. P.K., et. al., (1998), Reported the Nonalkloidal constituents of the seeds of *Gloriosa superbna lin..*
- Chauhan. S.K., et. al., (1998), Reported the development of HPTLC method from the estimation of colchicines in the different parts of *Gloriosa superba Linn..*

TISSUE CULTURE WORK

- Suganthi. C.P., et. al., (1993), Reported the effect of Rhizome extract of *Gloriosa superba Linn.*onAllium cepa.
- Samarajeewa. P.k., et. al., (1993), Reported the clonal propagation of the *Gloriosa superba Linn..*
- Yelne. M.B., et al, (1999), Reported the Invitro Propagation of *Gloriosa superba Linn.* Ane there advantages, disadvantages and constraints.
- Devagiri. G.M., et. al., (1999), Reported the Influence of hormone on rooting of *Gloriosa superba Linn.* Cuttings.
- Jadhav. S.Y., et. al., (2001), Reported the Somatic Embryogenesis and plant regeneration in *Gloriosa superba Linn..*
- Sivakumar. G., et. al., (2003), Reported the Embryoidogenesis and plant regeneration from leaf tissue of *Gloriosa superba Linn..*
- Somani. V.J., et. al., (1988), Reported the Invitro propagation and corm formation in *Gloriosa superba Linn..*

Chapter-3

AIM & PLAN OF WORK

AIM

To carried out standardization & pharmacological Evaluation of *Gloriosa superba Linn.* (Tubers).

PLAN OF WORK

- Botanical evaluation of the drug by microscopic and macroscopic examination.
- Standardization of plant part through following parameters.
    - Authentication
    - Effect of different chemical reagent on crude drug
    - Fluorescence analysis
    - Extractive values
    - Ash values
    - Loss on drying
    - Crude Fibre Contents
    - Foreign organic Matter.
    - Foaming Index
    - Swelling Index
    - Microbial determination
- Alcoholic extraction, Hydroalcoholic extraction & aqueous extraction of crude drug (Optimization of extract) by hot Soxhlet method.
- Preliminary phytochemical screening of different extract of the drug.

TLC/HPTLC FINGER PRINT PROFILE OF DIFFERENT EXTRACTS OF THE DRUG

- To Evaluation of Anti inflammatory activity of different extracts of the drug.
- To Evaluation of antimicrobial activity of different extracts of the drug.

Chapter-4
STANDARDIZATION

World Health Organization (WHO) currently encourages, recommends and promotes traditional herbal remedies in National Health care programs, because such drugs are easily available at low cost, are comparatively safe and reliable. Plant materials and herbal remedies derived from them represent a substantial proportion of the global drug market and thus internationally recognized guidelines for their quality assessment are necessary. The WHO emphasized the need to ensure quality control of medicinal plant products by using modern techniques and applying suitable standards.

For pharmaceutical purposes the quality of medicinal plant material must be as high as that of other medicinal preparations. However, it is impossible to assay for a specific chemical entity when the bioactive ingredient is not known. Further problem posed by those preparations which contain complex heterogeneous mixtures.

Directives on the analytical control of vegetable drug must take account of the fact that the material to be examined has complex and inconsistent composition. Therefore, the analytical limits can not be as precise as for the pure chemical compound. Vegetable drugs are inevitably inconsistent because of their composition and, hence, the standardization may be influenced by several factors such as age and origin, harvesting period, method of drying and so on. To eliminate some of the causes of inconsistency, one should use cultivated rather than wild plant which are often heterogeneous in respect of the above factors and consequently in their content of active principles.

The purpose of standardization of medicinal plant products is obviously to ensure therapeutic efficacy. Following parameters for standardization of raw materials have been prepared.

- Authentication
- Foreign matter
- Morphological studies
    - Macroscopic examination
    - Microscopical examination
- Volatile Matter
- Ash Value
- Extractive Values
- Loss on drying
- Chromatographic profile
- Pesticide Residue
- Determination of Heavy Metals
- Microbial Contamination
- Radioactive contamination.

The following parameters have been studied for the purpose of standardization of medicinal plant products.

BOTANICAL STANDARDS OF CRUDE DRUG

Procurement Of The Drug

The drug was procured from "G. M. Pharmacy" Bareilly(U.P). It is a renowned shop for the supply of crude drug. The drug was identified by Dr.Arvind Bhardwaj who is Botanist, Ghaziabad (U.P).

Macroscopy Of Drug (Tubers)

In case where the general appearance of the herb is similar to some other related species, a detailed study of the Morphological characters can be helpful in differentiating them. Macroscopical characters of *Gloriosa superba Linn.* (Tubers).

The Tubers are very long, solid,fleshy, cylindric,white yellowish in colour.

The Tubers are cylindrical or slightly flattened. The length of the tubers up to 15-25 cm long, and 2.5-4 cm thick. It is bifurcated in a"V"-Shaped in to two unequal limbs, pointed at both ends. Outer surface is brown, yellowish. Internally it is white and juicy. Fibers are present. Transversely cut dried pieces of root are oval in shape with a starchy and mealy white surface. These are up to 1 cm thick and 2 cm in diameter. It covered with a brown Epidermis on section white and starchy.

Fracture-tough and powdery: Odour- Slightly pungent: taste-mucilaginous slightly bitter & acrid, starch pure white and of a bitter taste. (Farooqi.A.A.et.al.,1993)

MICROSCOPY- Transverse section study of Gloriosa superba Linn.(Tuber)

The transverse section when seen in the microscope, the outer surface covered with brown Epidermis.

- **Epidermis-** It is made up of a single layer of parenchymatous cells. The cells are compactly arranged.The epidermal layer is covered by a thick layer of cuticle.
- **Cortex-** Next to the epidermis is a many layered cortex. The cortex is parenchymatous. The cells enclose small intercellular spaces. The endodermis is indistinguishable. The cells do not contain chloroplasts & are easily made out. The inner most layers of the cortex are non-green and can be designated as parenchymatous cortex. These cells contain starch grains and function as storage tissue.
- **Vascular bundles-**the vescular region is made up of distinct vascular bundles that are arranged in a ring.Vascular bundles are collateral with slight extensions on both sides of xylem. (Iyengar.M.A.,et. al.,2001; Vasishta.P.C.,1993)

POWDER MICROSCOPY OF *Gloriosa superba Linn.*(Tubers)

The powder of *Gloriosa superba Linn.* (Tubers) when seen under the microscope, different Cells observe in the powder.

- **Parenchyma** -The typical parenchymatous cells, which are either rounded or elongated, yellowish and are full of starch grains. Some of the parenchymatous cells are Opalescent.
- **Starch granules-**Characteristic,abundant, simple,ovoid or sack shaped, 5-60 microns in length and 3-30 microns in diameter.
- **Fibres-** The fibres are found in the single form not found in the groups the fibres are mostly non-lignified.
- **Calcium oxalate crystals-**present in the form of prisms, scattered all over in the powder. (Iyengar.M.A.,2001)

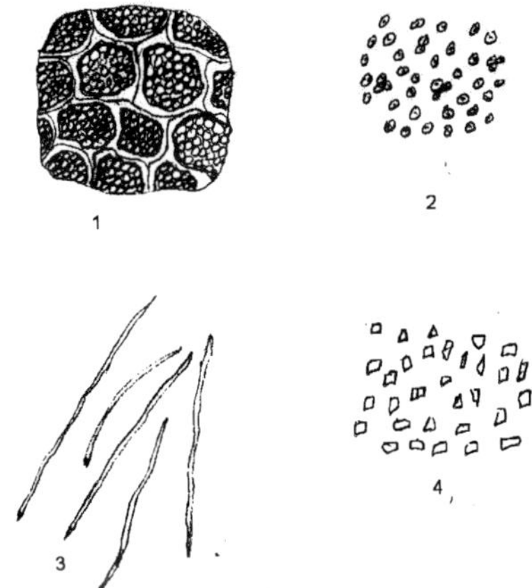

1. Parenchyma
2. Starch grains
3. Fibres
4. Calcium oxalate crystals

Fig-1: Microscopic character of powdered *Gloriosa superba Linn.* **(Tuber)**

PHYSICO-CHEMICAL STANDARDIZATION OF CRUDE DRUG

Effect of Different Chemical Reagent on Crude Drug Powder

Chemical tests of powder drug with different reagents were performed according to the method described by key, L.A. 1938. most of these tests were on colour identification of powder drug with specific substance. The observations were recorded in Table No.1.

Table No-1: Effect of different chemical reagents on crude drug powder of *Gloriosa superba Linn.* **(Tubers)**

S.No.	Treatment	Colour observed
1.	Conc. Hcl	Yellow
2.	Conc.HNO3	Dark Yellow
3.	Conc. H2SO4	Brown
4.	NaOH	Light yellow

S.No.	Treatment	Colour observed
5.	KOH	Light yellow
6.	Picric acid	Yellow
7.	Glacial acetic acid	Light yellow
8.	Tannic acid	Light brown
9.	Phloroglucinol+HCl	Orangish brown
10.	FeCl3	Dark yellow
11.	Iodine Solution	Light brown
12.	Saffron	Dark pink

Result- These were the characteristic test of *Gloriosa superba Linn.* (Tubers)

Fluorescence Analysis

Many herbs fluoresce when cut surface or powders are exposed to U.V. light and this can help in their identification. The powder drug was treated with different reagents and was examined under U.V. light (254 and 366nm).

The observed characteristics of *Gloriosa superba Linn.* (Tuber) were recorded in Table No.2. (Kay,L.A.,1938)

Table No-2: Fluorescence effect of different reagents on *Gloriosa superba Linn.* (Tubers) powder

S.No	Solvent	Observations	
		254 nm	366 nm
1.	Distilled water	Green black	White light black
2.	NaOH in methanol	Black	White black
3.	NaOH in water	Black	Dark black
4.	HNO_3	Clear	Dark black
5.	H_2SO_4	Clear	Dark brown
6.	HCL 50%	Clear	Brown
7.	HCL pure	Clear	Dark black

S.No	Solvent	Observations	
		254 nm	366 nm
8.	Acetone	Black	Whitish black
9.	Ethyl acetate	Black	White black
10.	Chloroform	Black	White black
11.	Pet. Ether	Clear	White

Result– There were the characteristic test of *Gloriosa superba Linn.*(Tubers).

Determination of Ash Value

The ash of any organic material is composed of their non-volatile inorganic components. Controlled incineration of crude drug results in an ash residue consisting of inorganic material (metallic salts and silica). This value varies within fairly wide limits and is, therefore, an important parameter for the purpose of evaluation of crude drugs. The ash value can be determined by three different methods to measure the total ash, the acid insoluble ash and the water soluble ash.

Determination of Total Ash

Total ash is designed to measure the total amount of material produced after complete incineration of the ground drug at as low as temperature as possible (about 450° C) to remove all the carbons. At higher temperature, the alkali chlorides may be volatile and may be lost by this process. The total ash usually consists of carbonates, phosphates, silicates and silica which includes both physiological ash – which is derived from the plant tissue itself and non-physiological ash- which is the residue of the adhering material to the plant, *e.g.*, sand and soil.

Indian Pharmacopoeia 1996 prescribes suitable methods for the determination of ash values. Method I for the crude vegetable drugs and Method II for the other substances.

Method I

Unless otherwise stated in the Individual monographs, weigh accurately 2-3 g of the air dried crude drug in the tarred platinum or silica dish and incinerate at a temperature not exceeding 450° C until free from carbon, cool and weigh. If a carbon free ash can not be obtained by this way, exhaust the charred mass in hot water, collect the residue on an ashless filter paper, incinerate the residue and filter paper until the ash is white or nearly white. Calculate the percentage of ash with reference to the air dried drug.

Method II

Heat the silica or platinum crucible to red hot for 30 minutes, allow to cool in a desiccator and weigh. Unless otherwise specified in the individual monograph, weigh accurately about 1 g of the substance being examined and evenly distribute in the crucible. Dry at 100° C to 105° C for 1 hr and ignite to constant weight in a muffle furnace at 600±25°C. Allow the crucible to cool in a desiccator after each ignition. The material should not catch fire in any time during the procedure. If after prolonged ignition a carbon free ash can not be obtained, proceed as directed in method I. Ignite to constant weight. Calculate the percentage of ash with reference to the air dried substance.

Acid Insoluble Ash

Ash insoluble in hydrochloric acid is the residue obtained after extracting the sulfated or total ash with HCl, calculate with reference to 100 g of drug. For the determination of acid insoluble ash as prescribed in IP 1996, method I is used unless otherwise directed in the Individual monograph.

Method I

Boil ash with 25 ml of 2M HCl for 5 minutes, collect the insoluble matter in a Gooch crucible or on an ash less filter paper, wash with hot water, ignite, cool in a desiccator and weigh. Calculate the percentage of acid insoluble ash with reference to the air dried drug.

Method II

Place the ash, as described or as directed in the individual monograph, in a crucible. Add 15 ml of water and 10 ml of hydrochloric acid, boil for 10 minutes and allow to cool. Collect the insoluble matter on an ash less filter paper, wash with hot water until the filtrate is neutral, ignite to dull redness, cool in a desiccator and weigh. Calculate the percentage of acid insoluble ash with reference to the air dried drug.

Water Soluble Ash

Water soluble ash is that part of the total ash content which is soluble in water. It is good indicator of either previous extraction of the water soluble salts in the drug or incorrect preparations. Thus, it is the difference in weight between the total ash and the residue obtained after treatment of Total ash with water.

As described in the IP 1996 to determine the water soluble ash, boil the ash as described before for 5 minutes with 25 ml of water. Collect the insoluble matter in a Gooch crucible or an ash less filter paper, wash with hot water and ignite for 15 minutes for a temperature not exceeding 450°C. Subtract the weight of the insoluble matter from the weight of the ash; the difference of weight represents the water soluble ash. Calculate the percentage of water soluble ash with reference to the air dried drug.

Table No-3: Ash Values of *Gloriosa superba Linn.* (Tubers)

S.No.	Total Ash (%)	Acid in Soluble Ash (%)	Water Soluble Ash (%)
1.	3.97	0.56	1.90
2.	4.23	0.55	1.75
3.	4.87	0.60	1.68
4.	3.85	0.50	1.61
Mean	4.23	0.55	1.73

Result- The total Ash values, Acid insoluble ash value and Water soluble ash value were found to be 4.23, 0.55, and 1.73, respectively.

Extractive Values

This method determines the amount of active constituents in a given amount of medicinal plant material when extracted with solvents. It is employed for that material for which no chemical on biological assay method exist. As mentioned in different official books (Indian pharmacopoeia 1996, British pharmacopoeia 1980, British Herbal Pharmacopoeia 1990 etc.), the determination of water-soluble and alcohol soluble extractives is used as a means of evaluating crude drugs which ate not readily estimated by other means.

Hot Extraction

Place about 10 gm of coarsely powdered air-dried material, accurately weighed, in a glass-stoppered conical flask. Add 10ml of water and weigh to obtain the total weight including the flask. Shake well and allow standing for 1 hour. Attach a reflux condenser to the flask and boil gently for 1 hour; cool and weigh Readjust to the original total weight with the solvent specified in the test procedure for the plant material concerned. Shake well and filter rapidly through a dry filter. Transfer 25ml of the filtrate to a tared flat-bottomed dish and evaporate to dryness on a coater-bath. Dry at 105^{0}C for 6 hours, cool in a desiccator for 30 minutes than weigh without delay. Calculate the content of extractable matter in mg per gm of air-dried material.

Table No-4: Hot alcoholic extractive value of ***Gloriosa superba Linn.*** **(Tubers)**

S.No.	Weight of empty dish (gm)	Weight of dish with extract (gm)	Weight of extract (gm)	Extractive value (%)
1.	45.2304	45.04757	0.2453	4.96
2.	42.1232	42.3875	0.2643	5.28
3.	48.3405	48.6237	0.2832	5.66
Mean	5.3			

Result – Hot alcoholic extractive value of *Gloriosa superba Linn.* (Tubers) was found to be 5.3%.

Table No-5: Hot Hydro alcoholic extractive value of ***Gloriosa superba Linn.*****(Tubers)**

S.No.	Weight of empty dish (gm)	Weight of dish with extract (gm)	Weight of extract (gm)	Extractive value (%)
1.	35.4323	35.8898	0.4575	9.15
2.	38.5532	39.0267	0.4735	9.47
3.	34.2562	34.7385	0.4823	9.64
Mean	**9.42**			

Result – Hot Hydro alcoholic extractive value of *Gloriosa superba Linn.* (Tubers) was found to be 9.42%.

Table No-6: Hot Aqueous extractive value of *Gloriosa superba Linn.* (Tubers)

S.No.	Weight of empty dish (gm)	Weight of dish with extract (gm)	Weight of extract (gm)	Extractive value (%)
1	45.2030	46.0123	0.8093	16.18
2	41.3060	42.1655	0.8595	17.19
3	46.2351	47.0737	0.8386	16.77
Mean	16.71			

Result – Hot Aqueous extractive value of *Gloriosa superba Linn.* (Tubers) was found to be 16.71%.

Cold Extraction

Place about 5.0gm of coarsely powdered air-dried material, accurately weighed, in a glass stoppered conical flask. Macerate with 100ml of the solvent specified for the plant material concerned for 6 hours, shaking frequently, and then allow standing for 18 hours. Filter rapidly taking care not to lose any solvent, transfer 25 ml of the filtrate to a tared flat-bottomed dish and evaporate to dryness on a water-bath. Dry at 105^{0}C for 6 hours, cool in a desiccator for 30 minutes and weigh without delay. Calculate the content of extractable matter in mg per gm of air-dried material.

Table No-7:- Cold alcoholic extractive value of *Gloriosa superba Linn.* (Tubers)

S.No.	Weight of empty dish (gm)	Weight of dish with extract (gm)	Weight of extract (gm)	Extractive value (%)
1	43.5689	43.6979	0.1290	2.58
2	42.4243	42.5623	0.1380	2.76
3	38.2532	38.3892	0.1360	2.72
Mean	2.68			

Result – Cold alcoholic extractive value of *Gloriosa superba Linn.* (Tubers) was found to be 2.68%.

Table No-8: Cold Hydro alcoholic extractive value of *Gloriosa superba Linn.* (Tubers)

S.No.	Weight of empty dish (gm)	Weight of dish with extract (gm)	Weight of extract (gm)	Extractive value (%)
1	33.4030	33.7625	0.3595	7.19
2	36.2015	36.5838	0.3782	7.56
3	40.0350	40.3470	0.3542	6.68
Mean	7.14			

Result – Cold Hydro alcoholic extractive value of *Gloriosa superba Linn.* (Tubers) was found to be 7.14%.

Table No-9: Cold Aqueous extractive value of *Gloriosa superba Linn.* (Tubers)

S.No.	Weight of empty dish (gm)	Weight of dish with extract (gm)	Weight of extract (gm)	Extractive value (%)
1	42.3202	42.7468	0.4266	8.53
2	44.2452	44.6824	0.4372	8.74
3	48.2351	48.7183	0.4832	9.66
Mean	8.97			

Result – Cold Aqueous extractive value of *Gloriosa superba Linn.* (Tubers) was found to be 8.97%.

Determination of Swelling Index

Many medicinal plant materials are of specific therapeutic or pharmaceutical utility because of their swelling properties, especially gums and those containing an appreciable amount of mucilage, pectin or hemicellulose.

The swelling index is the volume in ml taken up by the swelling of 1gm of plant material under specified conditions. Its determination is based on the addition of water or a swelling agent as specified in the test procedure for each individual plant material (either whole, cut or pulverized). Using a glass-stoppered measuring cylinder, the material is shaken repeatedly for 1 hour and then allowed to stand for a required period of time. The volume of the mixture (in ml) is then read.

The mixing of whole plant material with the swelling agent is easy to achieve, but cut or pulverized material requires vigorous shaking at specified intervals to ensure even distribution of the material in the swelling agent.

Procedure

Carry out simultaneously no fewer than three determinations for any given material. Introduce the specified quantity of the plant material concerned, previously reduced to the required fineness and accurately weighed, into a 25-ml glass-stoppered measuring cylinder. The internal diameter of the cylinder should be about 16mm, the length of the graduated portion about 125mm, marked in 0.2-ml divisions from 0 to 25ml in an upwards direction. Unless otherwise indicated in the test procedure, add 25ml of water and shake the mixture thoroughly every 10 minutes for 1 hour. Allow to stand for 3 hours at room temperature, or as specified. Measure the volume in ml occupied by the plant material, including any sticky mucilage. Calculate the mean value of the individual determinations, related to 1 g of plant material. (WHO; 2002)

Table No-10: Swelling index of *Gloriosa superba Linn.* **(Tubers)**

S.No.	Amount of Drug (gm)	Volume of water	Swelling Index
1.	1	25	1.9
2.	1	25	1.7
3.	1	25	1.8
Mean = 1.8 ml.			

Result- The swelling index of *Gloriosa superba Linn.*(Tubers) was found to be 1.8ml.

Foaming Index

Many medicinal plant materials contain saponins that can cause a persistent foam when an aqueous decoction is shaken. The foaming ability of an aqueous decoction of plant materials and their extracts is measured in terms of a foaming index.

Procedure

Reduce about 1 gm of the plant material to a coarse powder (sieve size no. 1250), weigh accurately and transfer to a 500-ml conical flask containing 100ml of boiling water. Maintain at moderate boiling for

30 sminutes. Cool and filter into a 100-ml volumetric flask and add sufficient water through the filter to dilute to volume.

Pour the decoction into 10 stoppered test-tubes (height 16cm, diameter 16mm) in successive portions of 1 ml, 2 ml, 3 ml, etc. up to 10ml, and adjust the volume of the liquid in each tube with water to 10ml. Stopper the tubes and shake them in a lengthwise motion for 15 seconds, two shakes per second. Allow to stand for 15 minutes and measure the height of the foam. The results are assessed as follows.

- If the height of the foam in every tube is less than 1cm, the foaming index is less than 100.
- If a height of foam of 1 cm is measured in any tube, the volume of the plant material decoction in this tube *(α)* is used to determine the index. If this tube is the first or second tube in a series, prepare an intermediate dilution in a similar manner to obtain a more precise result.
- If the height of the foam is more than 1 cm in every tube, the foaming index is over 1000. In this case repeat the determination using a new series of dilutions of the decoction in order to obtain a result. Calculate the foaming index using the following formula:

$$\frac{1000}{\alpha}$$

where α = the volume in ml of the decoction used for preparing the dilution in the tube where foaming to a height of 1 cm is observed. (WHO; 2002)

Table No-11: Foaming Index of *Gloriosa superba Linn.* **(Tubers)**

S.No	Number of test tubes	Foaming Index
1.	One	<100
2.	Two	<100
3.	Three	<100
4.	Four	<100
5.	Five	<100

S.No	Number of test tubes	Foaming Index
6.	Six	<100
7.	Seven	<100
8.	Eight	<100
9.	Nine	<100
10.	Ten	<100

Result:- The Foaming index of *Gloriosa superba Linn.* (Tubers) was found to be less than 100.

Foreign Organic Matter

Medicinal plant materials should be entirely free from visible signs of contamination by moulds or insects, and other animal contamination, including animal excreta. No abnormal odour, discoloration, slime or signs of deterioration should be detected. It is seldom possible to obtain marketed Plant materials that are entirely free from some form of innocuous foreign matter. However, no poisonous, dangerous or otherwise harmful foreign matter or residue should be allowed.

During storage, products should be kept in a clean and hygienic place, so that no contamination occurs. Special care should be taken to avoid formation of moulds, since they may produce aflatoxins.

Macroscopic examination can conveniently be employed for determining the presence of foreign matter in whole or cut plant materials. However, microscopy is indispensable for powdered materials.

Any soil, stones, sand, dust and other foreign inorganic matter must be removed before medicinal plant materials are cut or ground for testing. (WHO; 2002)

Procedure

- Weigh 100 gm of the sample (or the quantity specified in the monograph of the drug).
- Spread the sample on a white tile or a glass plate uniformly without overlapping.

- Inspect the sample with naked eyes or by means of a lens (5x or above).
- Separate the foreign organic matter (mentioned above) manually.
- After complete separation, weigh the matter and determine % w/w. present in the sample. (Khandelwal.K.R.,2002)

Result

- Drug sample taken =100gm
- Foreign organic matter = 4.85gm
- Percentage foreign organic matter= 4.85%

Crude Fibre Contents

Crude fibre is the residue of resistant tissues which can be obtained after giving treatment to the vegetable powder with dilute acid and alkali.

Advantages

- Determination of crude fibre is useful in distinguishing between similar drugs or in the detection of adulteration.
- It also helps to remove the more resistant parts of plant organs which can be used for microscopical examination.
- The process removes starch and other cell contents (cellulose is not affected if dilute reagents are used). It also destroys lignin present in the cell wall of lignified tissue.

Procedure

If crude drug contains appreciable amount of fat or oil, it must be removed first by extraction with suitable lipid solvent, before processing.

Weigh 2 grams of powdered drug in a beaker.

- Add 50 ml. of 10% v/v nitric acid.
- Heat to boil with constant stirring (till about 30 seconds after boiling starts).
- Strain through fine cotton cloth on a Buchner funnel.
- Give washing to the residue with boiling water. (Suction max be used),
- Transfer residue from the cloth to a beaker.

- Add 50 ml. of 2.5% v/v sodium hydroxide solution.
- Heat to boil. Maintain at boiling point for 30 seconds, stirring constantly.
- Strain and wash with hot water as mentioned earlier.
- For quantitative determination, transfer the residue in a cleaned and dried crucible,
- Weigh the residue and determine percentage crude fibres. For microscopical examination, residue is suspended in water or alcohol (70%) until required for use. (Khandelwal.K.R.,2002)

Table No-12: Crude fibre content in *Gloriosa superba Linn.* **(Tuber)**

S.No	Weight of powder drug (gm)	Weight of Empty china dish (gm)	Weight of China dish+Crude fibre (gm)	Weight of Crude fibre (gm)	Crude fibre (mg/gm)
1.	2	62.3268	62.4501	0.1233	61.65
2.	2	62.3268	62.4621	0.1353	67.65
3.	2	62.3268	62.4663	0.1395	69.75
4.	2	62.3268	62.4690	0.1422	71.1
Mean= 0.13507					

Result-The crude fiber content in *Gloriosa superba Linn.*(Tubers) was found to be 0.13507gm.

Loss On Drying

This parameter is used to determine the amount of moisture present in a particular sample.

Procedure

The powder drug (10 g) sample was placed on a tarred evaporating dish. The tarred evaporating dish is dried at 105°C for 6 hours and weighed. The drying was continued until two successive reading matches each other or the difference between two successive weighing was not more than 0.25% of constant weight.

The results of loss on drying are given in Tables-13.

Table No-13: Loss on drying in *Gloriosa superba Linn.* (Tubers) powder (10 g)

S. No.	Wt. of drug+Dish (Before drying) A (g)	Wt. Of drug+Dish (After drying) B (g)	A – B	Loss on Drying (%)
1.	65.432	65.152 65.205 65.205	0.227	2.27
2.	67.638	67.416	0.256	2.56
3.	63.588	67.382 67.382 63.338 63.318 63.318	0.270	2.70
Mean= 2.51				

Result- The loss on drying in *Gloriosa superba Linn.*(Tubers) was found to be 2.51%.

Determination of Microbial Counts

Microbial contamination in food, pharmaceuticals, beverages and herbal drug industries is of growing concern at all levels. Bacteria can grow in all kind of environment. The major damage takes place when bacteria grow in ready processed food, bulk drugs and injectables. It releases toxic substances, which act as an external antigen to immune system and the system does not have any defense mechanism to resist the same. This lead to several deleterious side effects and symptoms.

Medicinal plant materials generally carry a great number of bacteria and moulds. Current practices of harvesting, handling and production often causes additional contamination and microbial growth. There are some microbes seen in the plant materials that are pathogenic to the human beings, *e.g. Escharacia coli, Salmonella, Pseudomonus aureogenosae, Staphylococcus aureus*, and certain types of yeast and moulds. The presence of these microbes beyond certain limits causes several health hazards. Determination of microbial count is explained as per WHO guidelines.

Procedure

One gram of drug was taken and suspended in 50 ml of sterile distilled water. The suspension was shaken for sufficient period of time so as to allow maximum mixing. After this, the suspension was filtered by using a disposable sterilized filter paper. The filtrate was used as stock solution. Series dilution (1:1, 1:10, 1:100) of this stock solution were made and 1 ml of different diluted solutions was separately inoculated on nutrient agar medium and incubated at 37^{0}C for 24 hours.

After 24 hours, the Petri plates with most clearly visible colonies were taken and the number of colonies determined by using colony counter.

The microbial load per gram of sample was then calculated by using dilution factor.

Composition of Nutrient Agar Medium

1.	Yeast extract	0.3%
2.	Peptone	1%
3.	Agar	3 g
4.	Distilled water up to	100 ml
5.	pH	7 – 7.5

The pH was adjusted to 7.5 and autoclaved at 15 lbs per square inch pressure at 121^{0}C. The results are given in Table. 14.

Table No-14: Colony forming units on nutrient agar medium

Dilution of stock solution	Number of colonies		Colony characteristics	
	Drug	Control	Shape	Colour
1 in 1	Not Countable	Nil	Not clear	White
1 in 10	15	Nil	Circular	White
1 in 100	10	Nil	Circular	White

Drug – *Gloriosa superba Linn.*(Tubers powder)

Using the dilution factor, the number of colonies forming units per gram of drug was found to be 7.2 x 10^4 respectively.

Effect of UV radiation on the microbial count of the drug samples

To study the effect of sterilizing agent like UV radiation, the following exercise was performed. One gram of the drug was taken and kept under the laminar flow and exposure to UV radiation for a period of 12 hours. After 12 hours, a suspension of the exposed drugs was prepared by taking 50 ml of sterilized distilled water under aseptic conditions. The suspension was shaken sufficiently to allow maximum mixing. The suspension was then filtered using sterilized filter paper. The filtrate (1 ml) was separately inoculated on nutrient agar and incubated at 37^0 C for 24 hours. After the specified period of time, the plates were observed for the presence of colonies.

The result and observations are given in Table.15.

Table No-15: Effects of UV radiation on microbial growth

Sample	Colony observations	
	After 1 hr	After 12 hrs
Drug	2	No
Control	No	No

Drug – *Gloriosa superba Linn.* (Tubers powder)

Inference: On the basis of above experiment, it was found that exposure of drug to UV radiation for 12 hours completely removed any viable microorganisms and thus it could be used as a method to reduce the microbial load from the crude herbal drugs.

Chapter-5

PHYTOCHEMICAL STUDIES

COLLECTION & IDENTIFICATION OF PLANT MATERIAL

The drug was collected from "G.M. Pharmacy" Bareilly (U.P). It is a renowned shop for the supply of crude Drug. The Drug was identified by Dr.Arvind Bhardwaj who is Botanist Ghaziabad (U.P).

DRYING & SIZE REDUCTION

The Tubers of plant were dried in shade for the sufficient time. Then the size of the drug can be reduced to coarce powder. The powdered material was stored in airtight polythene pack

Extraction

Dried and powdered *Gloriosa superba Linn.* Tubers (250gm) were extracted with three different solvent, alcohol (99%), hydro alcohol (60:40), Aqueous, for 48 hours and gave about 35gm of Alcoholic, 40gm of hydro alcoholic and 45gm of aqueous extracts.(Sharma.A.K.,et.al.,1986)

These residues were vacuum evaporated to give brown residue.

Table No-16: Organoleptic characteristics of extracts of *Gloriosa superba Linn.*(Tubers)

S.No.	Parameters	Ethanolic Extract	Ethanol + water extract	Water extract
1.	Colour	Brown	Dark Brown	Dark Brown
2.	Odour	Characteristic	Characteristic	Characteristic
3.	Physical Appearance	Stickiness	Stickiness	Stickiness
4.	Extractive value	5.3	9.42	16.71

PRELIMINARY PHYTOCHEMICAL SCREENING

The preliminary phytochemical screening was carried out using the extracts for different types of chemical constituents. The qualitative chemical tests give the general idea regarding the nature of chemical constituents of crude drugs. The extracts were subjected to preliminary phytochemical investigation for detection of:

- Alkaloids
- Carbohydrates
- Glycosides
- Phenolic compounds
- Flavonoids
- Proteins and amino-acids
- Saponins
- Sterols
- Acidic compounds
- Mucilages

Tests for Alkaloids

Each of the extract residues was taken separately in 5 ml of 1.5 % hydrochloric acid and filtered. The filtrate was then tested with following reagents:

Dragendorff's Reagent

Few drops of Dragendorff's reagent were added in each of the extract and observed for formation of orange yellow precipitate.

Hager's Reagent

Few drops of Hager's reagent were added in each of the extract and observed for formation of yellow precipitate.

Wagner's Reagent

Few drops of Wagner's reagent were added in each of the extract and observed for formation of precipitate.

Mayer's Reagent

Few drops of Mayer's reagent were added in each of the extract and observed for formation of white or cream colored precipitate.

Test For Carbohydrates

Molisch's test

Treat the test solution with few drops of alcoholic alpha napthol. Add 0.2ml of con. Sulfuric acid slowly through the sides of the test tube, a purple to violet colour ring appears at the junction.

Benedict's test

Treat the test solution with few drops of Benedict's reagent (alkaline solution containing cupric citrate complex) and upon boiling on water bath, reddish brown precipitate forms if reducing sugars are present.

Barfoed's test

It is a general test for Monosaccharide. Heat the test tube containing 1ml of reagent and 1ml of solution of compound in a beaker of boiling water; if red cuprous oxide is formed within 2min, monosaccharide is present. **Disaccharide on** prolonged heating (about 10min) may also cause reduction, owing to partial hydrolysis to monosaccharides.

Camnelisation

Carbohydrates when treated with strong sulfuric acid, they undergo charring with the dehydration along with burning sugar smell.

Selwinoff's test

Hydrochloric acid reacts with ketose sugar to form derivatives of furfuraldehyde, which gives red colored compound when linked with resorcinol. Add compound solution to about 5ml of reagent and boil. Fructose give red color within half minute. The test is sensitive to 5.5mol / ltr if glucose is absent, but if glucose is present it is less sensitive and in addition of large amount of glucose can give similar color.

Tollen's test

To 100mg of compound add 2ml of Tollen's reagent and heat gently, a silver mirror is obtained inside the wall of the test tube, indicates the presence of aldose sugar.

Bromine water test

It gets decolorized by aldose but not by ketoses because bromine water oxidizes selectively the aldehyde group to carboxylic group, giving raise to general class of compounds called aldonic acid.

Fehling's test

Equal volume of Fehling's A (Copper sulfate in distilled water) and Fehling's B (Potassium tartarate and Sodium hydroxide in distilled water) reagents are mixed and few drops of sample is added and boiled, a brick red precipitate of cuprous oxide forms, if reducing sugars are present.

Tests for Glycosides

About 2 ml alcoholic extract were taken and subjected to the following tests:

Keller-Killiani Test

One ml of glacial acetic acid containing traces of ferric chloride and one ml of concentrated sulphuric acid were added to extract and observed for the formation of reddish brown colour at the junction of two layers and the upper layer turned bluish green in the presence of glycosides.

Borntrager's Test

One ml of benzene and 0.5 ml of dilute ammonia solution were added to the ethanolic extract and observed for the formation of reddish pink colour.

Legal Test

Concentrated ethanolic extracts were made alkaline with few drops of 10% sodium hydroxide solution and then freshly prepared sodium nitrosopruside solution was added to the solution and observed for formation of blue colour.

Baljet Test

To the concentrated ethanolic extracts sodium picrate reagent was added and observed for formation of orange or yellow colour.

Tests for Phenolic Compounds

Ferric chloride solution

The extracts were taken in water and warmed. To this 2 ml of ferric chloride solution was added and observed for formation of green or blue colour.

Lead acetate solution

To the extracts (2 ml) lead acetate solution was added and observed for formation of precipitate.

Gelatin solution

A few ml of gelatin solution was added to the aqueous extract and observed for formation of precipitate or turbidity.

Test For Flavonoids

Shinoda test (Magnesium Hydrochloride reduction test)

To the test solution add few fragments of Magnesium ribbon and add con. Hydrochloric acid drop wise, pink scarlet, crimson red or occasionally green to blue color appears after few minutes.

Zinc Hydrochloride reduction test

To the test solution add a mixture of Zinc dust and con. Hydrochloric acid. It gives red color after few minutes.

Alkaline reagent test

To the test solution add few drops of sodium hydroxide solution; formation of an intense yellow color which turns to colorless on addition of few drops of dil.acid indicates presence of Flavonoids.

Tests for Proteins and Amino-acids

Millon's Test

To few ml of alcoholic extract, five ml distilled water was added and filtered. To two ml of this filtrate 5-6 drops of Millon's reagent (solution of mercury nitrate and nitrous acid) were added and observed for formation of red precipitate.

Xanthoprotein Test

Two ml of extract few drops of nitric acid were added by the sides of the test tube and observed for formation of yellow colour.

Biuret Test

To the ammoniated alkaline filtrate of the extract 2-4 drops of 0.02 % copper sulphate solution were added and observed for formation of red or violet colour.

Ninhydrin Test

To the extract, lead acetate solution was added to precipitate tannins. The precipitate was spotted on a paper chromatogram, sprayed with ninhydrin reagent and heated at 110°C for 5 minutes and observed for formation of red or violet colour.

Tests for Saponins

a. **Foam Test:** Few mg of residue was taken in a test tube with a small amount of water and shaken vigorously for one minute and observed for formation of rich lather which was stable for more than ten minutes.

b. To the alcoholic extract few drops of sodium bicarbonate were added, shaken well, and observed for the formation of honey comb like frothing.

Tests for Sterols

The alcoholic extract was evaporated to dryness and the residue was extracted with petroleum ether and acetone. The insoluble residue left after extraction with petroleum ether and acetone was tested for sterols as:

Liebermann-Buchard Test

The insoluble residue was dissolved in chloroform and few drops of acetic anhydride were added along with a few drops of concentrated sulphuric acid from the sides of the test tube and observed for the formation of blue to blood red colour.

Salkowski Reaction

To the extract two ml of concentrated sulphuric acid were added and observed for the formation of yellow ring at the junction which turn red after one minute.

Herche's Reaction

To the residue 2-3 ml of trichloroacetic acid were added, heated, and observed for the formation of red to violet colour.

Tests for Acidic compounds

To the alcoholic extract sodium bicarbonate solution was added and observed for the production of effervescences.

A small amount of alcoholic extract was taken in warm water and filtered. The filtrate was then tested with litmus paper and methyl orange and observed for the appearance of blue colour.

Tests for Mucilage

The extract was treated with ruthenium red solution in lead acetate and observed for the formation of pink colour. (Khandelwal..K.R.,2002; Kokate.C.K.et.al.,2001)

Table No-17: Results were obtained after the preliminory Phytochemical screening of different extracts of *Gloriosa superba Linn.* (Tubers)

S.No.	Constituent	Tests	Alc. Ext.	Hyd. Alc. Ext.	Aque. Ext
1.	Alkaloids	i. Mayer's test	+	+	+
		ii. Dragen droff's test	+	+	-
		iii.Wagner's test	+	+	-
		iv. Hager's test	+	+	-
2.	Carbohydrates	i. Molish's test	+	+	+
		ii. Benedicts test	+	+	+
		iii. Barfoed's test	-	-	-
		iv. Fehling's test	-	-	+
		v. Tollen's phloroglucinol test	+	+	-
		vi. Iodine test	-	-	-
		vii. Tannec acid test	-	+	+

S.No.	Constituent	Tests	Alc. Ext.	Hyd. Alc. Ext.	Aque. Ext
3.	Glycoside's	i. Keller- Killiani test	+	+	-
		ii. Legal's test	-	-	-
		iii. Borntrager's test	-	-	-
		iv. Modified B.T. test	-	-	-
		v. Saponin (Foam) test	-	+	+
4.	Tannins and phenolic compounds	-2-3 ml of Extracts + fewdrops of following reagent			
		5% $FeCl_3$ Solution	-	-	-
		Lead Acetate solution	+	+	+
		$K_2Cr_2O_7$ Solution	-	-	-
		Acetic acid Solution	-	-	-
		Dilute HNO_3	-	-	-
		Bromine water	-	-	-
5.	Amino Acids	Ninhydrin test	+	+	+
		Tyrosine test	-	+	-
		Cysteine test	-	-	-
6.	Proteins	Biuret test	-	-	-
		Millon's test	-	-	-
		Xantho protein test	-	-	-
		Sulphur test	-	+	-
		Precipitation test			
		• Absolute alcohol	-	-	-
		• 5% Hg Cl_2 Solution	-	-	-
		• 5% Cu So_4	-	-	+
		• 5% Lead acetate	+	-	+
		• 5%ammonium	+	-	-
		• Sulphate			

S.No.	Constituent	Tests	Alc. Ext.	Hyd. Alc. Ext.	Aque. Ext
7.	Flavonoids	Shinoda test	-	-	-
		Lead Acetate test	+	+	-
		Sodium hydroxide test	-	-	+
8.	Organic Acid	This test only for Aqueous extract of drug			
		Oxalic acid			+
		Tartaric acid			-
		Citric acid			+
		Malic acid			-
9.	Steroid	Salkowski reaction	+	+	+
10.	Volatile oils	After distillation			
		• Filter paper test	-	-	-
		• Odour test	-	-	-
		• Solubility test	-	-	-

+ = Present, - = Absent

Optimization of the extract

This is the method to measure the optimum time for the complete extraction of herbal drug. Optimization of *Gloriosa superba Linn.* were carried out by solvents: Aqueous, Hydro-alcoholic & alcoholic. The observations were recorded in Table- 18,19&20.

Method

Drug powder (10gm) was extracted in a Soxhlet apparatus, using different solvents. After two hours, the extract was separated, evaporated to dryness and weighed. After two hour weight of dried extract was noted. This process was continued till the extract obtained was of negligible amount.

Table No-18: Alcoholic optimization of extract of *Gloriosa superba Linn.* (Tubers)

Hours	Initial Wt.of China dish(gm)	Final Wt.of China dish (gm)	Wt. Of Residue (gm)
2	48.21	49.85	1.64
4	48.21	49.15	0.94
6	48.21	48.88	0.67
8	48.21	48.645	0.435
10.	48.21	48.479	0.269
12	48.21	48.357	0.147
14	48.21	48.30	0.09

Result- It took 14 hrs for the optimization of Alcoholic extract of *Gloriosa superba Linn.* (Tubers).

Table No-19: Hydro alcoholic optimization of extract ethanol : water (60 :40) of *Gloriosa superba Linn.* (Tubers)

Hours	Initial Wt.of China dish(gm)	Final Wt.of China dish (gm)	Wt. Of Residue (gm)
2	48.21	50.13	1.92
4	48.21	49.22	1.01
6	48.21	49.10	0.89
8	48.21	48.88	0.67
10.	48.21	48.64	0.43
12	48.21	48.49	0.28
14	48.21	48.40	0.19
16	48.21	48.31	0.10
18	48.21	48.28	0.07
20	48.21	48.24	0.03

Result- It took 20 hrs for the optimization of Hydro alcoholic extract of *Gloriosa superba Linn.* (Tubers).

Table No-20: Aqueous Optimization of Extract of *Gloriosa superba Linn.*(Tubers)

Hours	Initial Wt.of China dish(gm)	Final Wt.of China dish (gm)	Wt. Of Residue (gm)
2	48.21	51.03	2.82
4	48.21	49.67	1.46
6	48.21	49.18	0.97
8	48.21	48.99	0.78
10.	48.21	48.79	0.58
12	48.21	48.60	0.39
14	48.21	48.50	0.29
16	48.21	48.41	0.20
18	48.21	48.36	0.15
20	48.21	48.32	0.11
22	48.21	48.29	0.08
24	48.21	48.27	0.06

Result- It took 24 hrs for the optimization of Aqueous extract of *Gloriosa superba Linn.* (Tubers).

Table No-21: The Results were obtained after the phytochemical screening of alcoholic extract of *Gloriosa superba Linn.* (Tubers) at different time interval of the extraction(After Successive extraction)

S.No.	Constituent	Tests	2hr	4hr	6hr	8hr	10hr	12hr
1.	Alkaloids	i. Mayer's test	+	+	+	+	-	-
		ii. Dragen droff's test	+	+	+	-	-	-
		iii. Wagner's test	+	+	+	+	-	-
		iv. Hager's test	+	+	+	-	-	-
2.	Carbohydrates	i. Molish's test	+	+	+	+	+	-
		ii. Benedicts test	+	+	-	-	-	-
		iii. Barfoed's test	-	-	-	-	-	-
		iv. Fehling's test	-	-	-	-	-	-
		v. Tollen's phloroglucinol test	+	+	-	-	-	-
		vi. Iodine test	-	-	-	-	-	-
		vii. Tannec acid test	-	-	-	-	-	-

S.No.	Constituent	Tests	2hr	4hr	6hr	8hr	10hr	12hr
3.	Glycoside's	i.Keller- Killiani test	+	+	-	-	-	-
		ii. Legal's test	-	-	-	-	-	-
		iii. Borntrager's test	-	-	-	-	-	-
		iv. Modified B.T. test	-	-	-	-	-	-
		v. Saponin (Foam) test	-	-	-	-	-	-
4.	Tannins and phenolic compounds	-2-3 ml of Extracts + fewdrops of following reagent						
		5% $FeCl_3$ Solution	-	-	-	-	-	-
		Lead Acetate solution	+	+	-	-	-	-
		$K_2Cr_2O_7$ Solution	-	-	-	-	-	-
		Acetic acid Solution	-	-	-	-	-	-
		Dilute HNO_3	-	-	-	-	-	-
		Bromine water	-	-	-	-	-	-
5.	Amino Acids	Ninhydrin test	+	+	+	+	-	-
		Tyrosine test	-	-	-	-	-	-
		Cysteine test	-	-	-	-	-	-
6.	Proteins	Biuret test	-	-	-	-	-	-
		Millon's test	-	-	-	-	-	-
		Xantho protein test	-	-	-	-	-	-
		Sulphur test	-	-	-	-	-	
		Precipitation test						

S.No.	Constituent	Tests	2hr	4hr	6hr	8hr	10hr	12hr
		• Absolute alcohol	-	-	-	-	-	-
		• 5% Hg Cl_2 Solution	-	-	-	-	-	-
		5% Cu So_4	-	-	-	-	-	-
		5% Lead acetate	+	+	-	-	-	-
		5%ammonium Sulphate	+	+	-	-	-	-
7.	Flavonoids	Shinoda test	-	-	-	-	-	-
		Lead Acetate test	+	+	-	-	-	-
		Sodium hydroxide test	-	-	-	-	-	-
8.	Organic Acid	This test only for Aqueous extract of drug.						
		Oxalic acid						
		Tartaric acid						
		Citric acid						
		Malic acid						
9.	Steroid	Salkowski reaction	+	+	+	+	-	-
10.	Volatile oils	After distillation						
		Filter paper test	-	-	-	-	-	-
		Odour test	-	-	-	-	-	-
		Solubility test	-	-	-	-	-	-

hr= Hours
(+) = Present, (-) = Absent

Table No-22: The Results were obtained after the phytochemical screening of Hydroalcoholic extract of *Gloriosa superba Linn.* (Tubers) at different time interval of the extraction (After Successive extraction)

S.No.	Constituent	Tests	2hr	4hr	6hr	8hr	10hr	12hr
1.	Alkaloids	i. Mayer's test	+	+	+	-	-	-
		ii. Dragen droff's test	+	+	+	-	-	-
		iii. Wagner's test	+	+	+	+	-	-
		iv. Hager's test	+	+	+	-	-	-
2.	Carbohydrates	i. Molish's test	+	+	+	+	+	-
		ii. Benedicts test	+	+	+	+	+	-
		iii. Barfoed's test	-	-	-	-	-	-
		iv. Fehling's test	-	-	-	-	-	-
		v. Tollen's phloroglucinol test	+	+	-	-	-	-
		vi. Iodine test	-	-	-	-	-	-
		vii. Tannec acid test	+	+	-	-	-	-
3.	Glycoside's	i.Keller- Killiani test	+	+	-	-	-	-
		ii. Legal's test	-	-	-	-	-	-
		iii. Borntrager's test	-	-	-	-	-	-
		iv. Modified B.T. test	-	-	-	-	-	-
		v. Saponin (Foam) test	+	+	+	-	-	-
4.	Tannins and phenolic compounds	-2-3 ml of Extracts + fewdrops of following reagent						
		5% $FeCl_3$ Solution	-	-	-	-	-	-
		Lead Acetate solution	+	+	+	+	+	-
		$K_2Cr_2O_7$ Solution	-	-	-	-	-	-
		Acetic acid Solution	-	-	-	-	-	-
		Dilute HNO_3	-	-	-	-	-	-
		Bromine water	-	-	-	-	-	-

S.No.	Constituent	Tests	2hr	4hr	6hr	8hr	10hr	12hr
5.	Amino Acids	Ninhydrin test	+	+	+	+	+	-
		Tyrosine test	+	+	-	-	-	-
		Cysteine test	-	-	-	-	-	-
6.	Proteins	Biuret test	-	-	-	-	-	-
		Millon's test	-	-	-	-	-	-
		Xantho protein test	-	-	-	-	-	-
		Sulphur test	+	+	-	-	-	-
		Precipitation test						
		• Absolute alcohol	-	-	-	-	-	-
		• 5% Hg Cl_2 Solution	-	-	-	-	-	-
		• 5% Cu So_4	-	-	-	-	-	-
		• 5% Lead acetate	-	-	-	-	-	-
		• 5%ammonium Sulphate	-	-	-	-	-	-
7.	Flavonoids	Shinoda test	-	-	-	-	-	-
		Lead Acetate test	+	+	-	-	-	-
		Sodium hydroxide test	-	-	-	-	-	-
8.	Organic Acid	This test only for Aqueous extract of drug.						
		Oxalic acid						
		Tartaric acid						
		Citric acid						
		Malic acid						
9.	Steroid	Salkowski reaction	+	+	+	+	+	-
10.	Volatile oils	After distillation						
		Filter paper test	-	-	-	-	-	-
		Odour test	-	-	-	-	-	-
		Solubility test	-	-	-	-	-	-

hr = Hours

+ = presents, - = Absant

Table No-23: The result were obtained after the phytochemical screening of Aqueous extract of *Gloriosa superba Linn.* (Tubers) at different time interval of the extraction (After Successive extraction)

S.No.	Constituent	Tests	2hr	4hr	6hr	8hr	10hr	12hr
1.	Alkaloids	i. Mayer's test	+	+	+	-	-	-
		ii. Dragen droff's test	-	-	-	-	-	-
		iii. Wagner's test	-	-	-	-	-	-
		iv. Hager's test	-	-	-	-	-	-
2.	Carbohydrates	i. Molish's test	+	+	+	+	+	-
		ii. Benedicts test	+	+	+	-	-	-
		iii. Barfoed's test	-	-	-	-	-	-
		iv. Fehling's test	+	+	-	-	-	-
		v. Tollen's phloroglucinol test	-	-	-	-	-	-
		vi. Iodine test	-	-	-	-	-	-
		vii. Tannec acid test	+	+	-	-	-	-
3.	Glycoside's	i.Keller- Killiani test	-	-	-	-	-	-
		ii. Legal's test	-	-	-	-	-	-
		iii. Borntrager's test	-	-	-	-	-	-
		iv. Modified B.T. test	-	-	-	-	-	-
		v. Saponin (Foam) test	+	+	+	+	+	-
4.	Tannins and phenolic compounds	-2-3 ml of Extracts + fewdrops of following reagent						
		5% $FeCl_3$ Solution	-	-	-	-	-	-
		Lead Acetate solution	+	+	+	+	-	-
		$K_2Cr_2O_7$ Solution	-	-	-	-	-	-
		Acetic acid Solution	-	-	-	-	-	-
		Dilute HNO_3	-	-	-	-	-	-
		Bromine water	-	-	-	-	-	-
5.	Amino Acids	Ninhydrin test	+	+	+	-	-	-
		Tyrosine test	-	-	-	-	-	-
		Cysteine test	-	-	-	-	-	-

6.	Proteins	Biuret test	-	-	-	-	-	-
		Millon's test	-	-	-	-	-	-
		Xantho protein test	-	-	-	-	-	-
		Sulphur test	-	+	-	-	-	-
		Precipitation test	-	-	-	-	-	-
		• Absolute alcohol	-	-	-	-	-	-
		• 5% Hg Cl_2 Solution	-	-	-	-	-	-
		• 5% Cu So_4	+	+	-	-	-	-
		• 5% Lead acetate	+	+	+	-	-	-
		• 5%ammonium	-	-	-	-	-	-
		•Sulphate	-	-	-	-	-	-
7.	Flavonoids	Shinoda test	-	-	-	-	-	-
		Lead Acetate test	-	-	-	-	-	-
		Sodium hydroxide test	+	+	+	+	-	-
8.	Organic Acid	This test only for Aqueous extract of drug.	+	+	-	-	-	-
		Oxalic acid	-	-	-	-	-	-
		Tartaric acid	-	-	-	-	-	-
		Citric acid	+	+	-	-	-	-
		Malic acid	-	-	-	-	-	-
9.	Steroid	Salkowski reaction	+	-	-	-	-	-
10.	Volatile oils	After distillation	-	-	-	-	-	-
		Filter paper test	-	-	-	-	-	-
		Odour test	-	-	-	-	-	-
		Solubility test						

hr = Hours

+ = presents, - = Absant

Chapter-6

CHROMATOGRAPHIC PROFILE

Thin layer chromatographic (TLC) studies were carried out for alcoholic, hydroalcoholic and aqueous extracts to confirm the presence of the phytoconstituents detected in qualitative chemical tests and to know how many compounds are present in them.

TLC is mode of chromatography in which sample is applied as a small spot or to the origin of a thin absorbent layer supported on a glass, plastic or metal plate. The mobile phase moves through stationary phase by capillary action, sometimes assisted by gravity or pressure. TLC separation takes place in the open layers with each component having the same total migration time but different migration distances. Mobile phase consists of a single solvent or mixture of solvent. Numerous fixed absorbents have been used, including Silica gel, Cellulose, Polyamide, Alumina, Ion exchanger and Chemically bonded Silica gel.

The stationary phase of the TLC are prepared using various techniques such as pouring, dipping and spraying. However ready made prepared stationary phase (TLC plates) are also available in the market. The prepared plates are allowed for setting (air drying). This is done to avoid cracks on the surface of adsorbent. After setting the plates are activated by keeping in an oven at 100 - 120^{0}C for 1hr. activation of TLC plates is nothing but removing water / moisture and other adsorbed substances from the surface of any adsorbent, by heating at high temperature so that adsorbent activity is retained. (Wagner,H.et.al., 2002; Egon stahl. 2005)

THIN LAYER CHROMATOGRAPHY OF DIFFERENT EXTRACTS OF GLORIOSA SUPERBA LINN. (TUBERS)

The active extracts under study were subjected to thin layer chromatography to find out the number of components present in it.

a. **Preparation of the Plate-** The adsorbent used for preparation of thin layer plates (TLC) as stationary phase was silica gelG. Silica gel G (25g) in distilled water (35ml) was allowed to swell for about 15-20 min in a glass mortar until it become homogeneous. Additional 15ml of distilled water was added with stirring. The silica gel G suspension was spread with a spreader on thin layer chromatographic plates. The prepared plates were air-dried and activated in an oven at 110^{0}C for 30 minutes. The activated plates were stored in a desiccator. (Chauhan, S.K.,et al, 1998)

b. **Application of Sample-** For applying test samples on plate, glass capillaries were used. The distance of minimum 1 cm was kept between two spots. The spots were marked on the top of the plate to know their identity.

c. **Chromatographic Chamber & Development of Chromatogram-** Chromatographic rectangular glass chamber was used in the experiment. To avoid insufficient chamber saturation and the undesirable edge effect a smooth filter paper approximately 15 X 40 cm was placed in the chromatographic chamber (in a "U" shape) and soaked in the solvent development was allowed to proceed until the solvent front has been traveled the required distance (usually 10-15cm), then the plate was removed from the chamber and solvent font was immediately marked with a pointer object. The plate was dried using heat on a current of air as appropriate. The experiments were carried out at room temperature in diffused daylight.

d. **Solvent System-** Number of solvent system were tried, the solvent systems with satisfactory resolution and useful are given in table. (Chauhan. S.K.,et.al.,1998; Thakur.R.S.,et.al.,1975)

e. **Spray reagents-** Spray reagents used for visualizing components on chromatogram are dragendorff reagent/$NaNo_2$. The Rf value was calculated as follows: (Mukherjee. P.K., 2000; Chaudhuri. P.K., et.al., 1993)

$$Rf = \frac{\text{Distance traveled by the sample.}}{\text{Distance traveled by the solvent.}}$$

Table No-24: TLC Profile of different extracts of *Gloriosa superba Linn.* (Tubers) in different solvent system

S.No.	Test Sample	Solvent system	No. of Spots	Resolution
1.	Ethanolic extract	-Ethyl acetate : Methanol : water (77:13.5:8) - Ethyl acetate : Formic Acid : Glacial Acetic acid : water (100:11:11:27)	2 4	Good Fair
		-Ethyl acetate: Methanol: water (100:13.5:10) -Chloroform:Acetone(1:1)	4. 3.	Fair Good
		-Toluene :Ethyl acetate :Methanol :Acetic acid(60:30:10:10) -Toluene :Ethyl acetate:Acetic acid(60:40:10)	3 2	Fair Good
2.	Ethanol+Water Extract	-Ethyl acetate :Formic acid :Glacial acetic acid :Water(100:11:11:27) -Ethyl acetate :Methanol :Water(90:10:10)	4 2	Fair Good
		-Ethyl acetate :Methanol :Water(100:13.5:10) -Chloroform :Acetone(1:1)	4 2	Fair Good
		-Toluene :Ethyl acetate :Methanol :Acetic acid(60:30:10:10) -Ethyl acetate :Methanol :Water(77:13.5:8)	3 2	Fair Good
3	Water Extract	-Ethyl acetate :Methanol :Water(77:13.5:8) -Ethyl acetate :Formic acid :Glacial acetic acid :Water(100:11:11:27)	2 3	Good Fair
		-Ethyl acetate :Methanol :Water(100:13.5:10) -Chloroform :Acetone(1:1)	3 2	Fair Good
		-Ethyl acetate :Methanol :Water(90:10:10) -Toluene :Ethyl acetate :Acetic acid(60:40:10)	3 2	Fair Good

Adsobent- Activated Silica gel-G, Detecting Agent- Iodine

Result- The different Extracts of *Gloriosa superba Linn.*(Tubers) showed different spots on TLC, which indicate the number of constituents present in different extracts.

HIGH PERFORMANCE THIN LAYER CHROMATOGRAPHY OF DIFFERENT EXTRACT OF GLORIOSA SUPERBA LINN. (TUBERS)

1. **Selection of Solvent System-** HPTLC of different Extracts of *Gloriosa superba Linn.* (Tubers) was carried out by using the different solvent system shown in the table. (Chauhan, S.K., et al, 1998;Wagner, H. et. al., 2002)
2. **Application of Sample-** A small quantity of different extracts (3mg) was dissolved in different extracting solvents (1ml) and 10 m l sample was applied on precoated plate with the help of linomat IV applicator.
3. **Development of Chromatogram-** A rectangular twin trough glass chamber was used in the experiment. To avoid in sufficient chamber saturation and the undesirable edge effect, a smooth filter paper was placed in the glass chamber and was allowed to be soaked in the developing solvent. The moistened paper was pressed against the walls of the chamber so that it adheres to the walls. The chamber was allowed to saturate for 15 min, before use. The experiment was carried out at room temperature in diffused daylight.

Procedure

The plate was dipped in a saturated chromatographic chamber containing the solvent system and was allowed the elute upto 8cm and was air-dried. The spot were scanned in CAMAG TLC scanner-3 in Courtesy to Toxicology Lab, IVRI, Izatnagar, Bareilly (U.P), India. (Chauhan.S.K.,et.al.,1998)

Chromatographic Condition

Following are the chromatographic conditions required to get an effective resolutions by selected mobile phase.

Stationary phase	:	HPTLC precoated, silica gel 60 F254 (Merck)
Size	:	5 X 10 Cm
Developing Chamber	:	Twin trough glass chamber

Mode of application	:	Band
Band Size	:	5 mm
Separation technique	:	Ascending
Temperature	:	20-25^{0}C
Saturation time	:	15 min
Scanning wavelength	:	260 nm, 254nm
Scanning mode	:	Absorbance/Reflectance.

(Stahl, E. 1965)

Table No-25: High performance thin layer chromatography of different extracts of *Gloriosa superba Linn.*(Tubers) in different solvent system

S.No.	Test Extract	Solvent System	No. of spots in Camag Scanner	Rf values
1	Ethonolic Extract	Ethyl acetate:Methanol:Water (100:13.5:10)	5	0.19, 0.37, 0.43, 0.50, 0.85
2	Ethanolic + Water Ext.	Ethyl acetate:Methanol:Water (100:13.5:10)	7	0.08, 0.15, 0.37, 0.43, 0.49,0.73, 0.83.
3	Water Extract	Ethyl acetate:Methanol:Water (100:13.5:10)	5	0.10, 0.18, 0.42, 0.47, 0.82

S.No.	Test Extract	Solvent System	No. of spots in Camag Scanner	Rf values
1	Ethonolic Extract	Ethyl acetate: Glacial acetic acid: Formic Acid: Water (100:11:11:27)	7	0.04, 0.12, 0.14,0.22, 0.32,0.47,0.56.
2	Ethanolic + Water Ext.	Ethyl acetate: Glacial acetic acid: Formic Acid: Water (100:11:11:27)	5	0.03, 0.06,0.34,0.45,0.56.

S.No.	Test Extract	Solvent System	No. of spots in Camag Scanner	Rf values
3	Water Extract	Ethyl acetate: Glacialacetic acid:FormicAcid: Water (100:11:11:27)	3	0.03, 0.11,0.16.

Result– The different Extracts of *Gloriosa superba Linn.* (Tubers) showed different spots in CAMAG SCANNER, which indicate the number of constituent present in different extracts. The Rf values of these spots were calculated which were showed in Table.25.

winCATS Planar Chromatography Manager

Toxicology Lab,
IVRI, Izatnagar, Bareilly,
UP, India

Analysis Report

SOP document	
Validated	Design
Description :	
Analysis	C:\CAMAG\winCATS\Data\Extr-II G. superba.cna
Created/used by	Supervisor Tuesday, April 18, 2006 11:33:28 AM
Current user	Supervisor

Detection - CAMAG TLC Scanner 3

Information

Application position	15.0 mm
Solvent front position	80.0 mm

Instrument	CAMAG TLC Scanner 3 "Scanner3_120716" S/N 120716 (1.14.22)
Executed by	Supervisor Tuesday, April 18, 2006 11:33:10 AM
Number of tracks	5
Position of first track X	10.3 mm
Distance between tracks	20.0 mm
Scan start pos. Y	11.4 mm
Scan end pos. Y	90.0 mm
Slit dimensions	6.00 x 0.45 mm, Micro
Optimize optical system	Light
Scanning speed:	20 mm/s
Data resolution:	100 µm/step

Measurement Table

Wavelength	254
Lamp	D2
Measurement Type	Remission
Measurement Mode	Absorption
Optical filter	Second order
Detector mode	Automatic
PM high voltage	288 V

Integration

Properties

Data filtering	Savitsky-Golay 7
Baseline correction	Lowest Slope
Peak threshold min. slope	5
Peak threshold min. height	10 AU
Peak threshold min. area	50
Peak threshold max. height	990 AU
Track start position	15.0 mm
Track end position	89.9 mm
Display scaling	Automatic

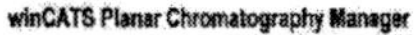

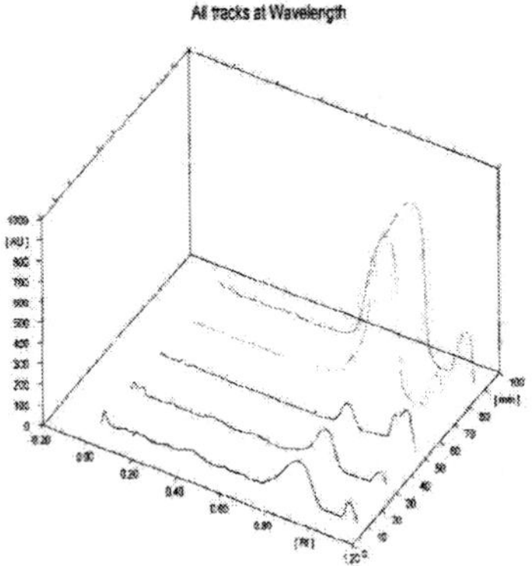

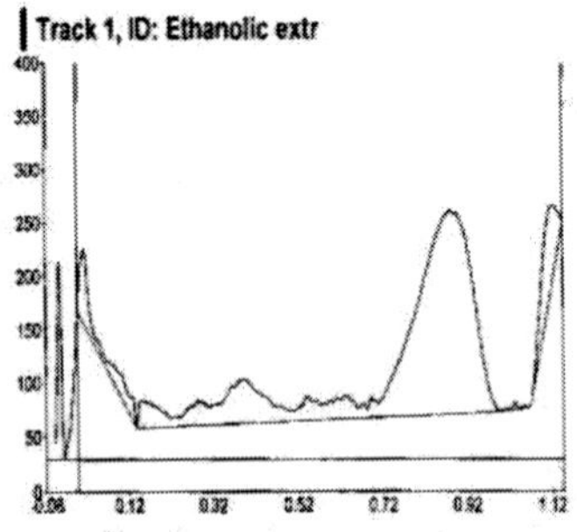

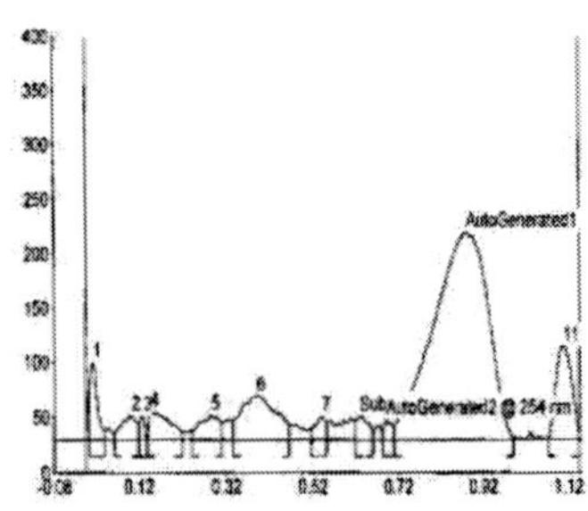

Peak	Start Rf	Start Height	Max Rf	Max Height	Max %	End Rf	End Height	Area	Area %	Assigned sSubstance
1	0.01	53.0	0.02	70.4	13.11	0.04	8.1	894.0	3.23	unknown*
2	0.07	6.0	0.11	21.9	4.09	0.12	15.6	593.3	2.14	unknown*
3	0.12	16.1	0.13	21.1	3.92	0.14	0.6	181.2	0.65	unknown*
4	0.14	5.9	0.15	24.7	4.60	0.22	7.4	914.9	3.30	unknown*
5	0.25	7.9	0.29	22.4	4.18	0.32	15.4	766.0	2.77	unknown*
6	0.34	18.2	0.39	39.7	7.40	0.47	13.8	2423.4	8.75	unknown*
7	0.52	9.7	0.55	21.4	3.98	0.56	16.4	397.3	1.43	unknown*
8	0.62	17.1	0.63	21.4	3.98	0.66	8.1	445.9	1.61	Substance 1
9	0.69	7.3	0.70	18.1	3.98	0.71	11.9	253.8	0.92	AutoGenerated2
10	0.72	12.2	0.89	190.1	35.43	1.00	2.0	18482.7	66.73	AutoGenerated1
11	1.08	0.9	1.11	85.4	15.92	1.15	4.6	2343.1	8.46	unknown*

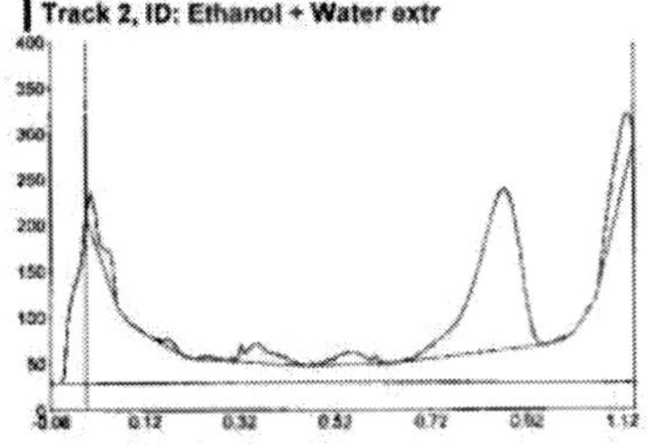

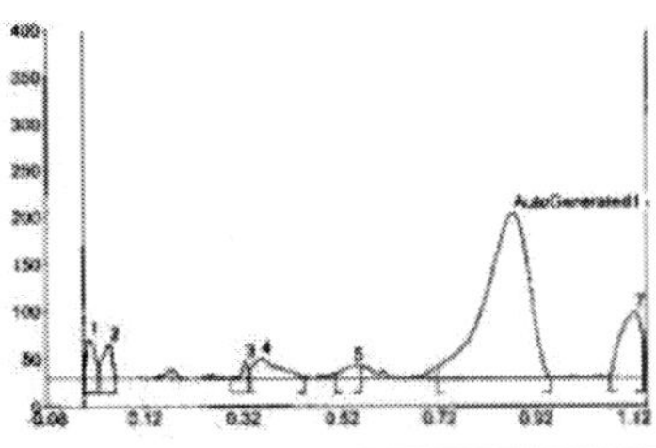

Peak	Start Rf	Start Height	Max Rf	Max Height	Max %	End Rf	End Height	Area	Area %	Assigned Substance
1	0.00	7.0	0.01	42.2	11.23	0.03	14.9	538.5	3.26	unknown*
2	0.03	15.0	0.05	36.5	9.71	0.06	0.8	552.1	3.35	unknown*
3	0.30	0.1	0.33	18.2	4.84	0.34	9.2	149.3	0.90	unknown*
4	0.34	9.5	0.36	21.2	5.61	0.45	1.3	837.6	5.08	unknown*
5	0.51	5.1	0.55	13.3	3.54	0.56	12.5	357.5	2.17	unknown*
6	0.72	12.3	0.88	174.9	46.51	0.96	0.3	11884.6	72.02	AutoGenerated1
7	1.08	0.8	1.13	69.8	18056	1.15	38.4	2182.2	13.22	unknown*

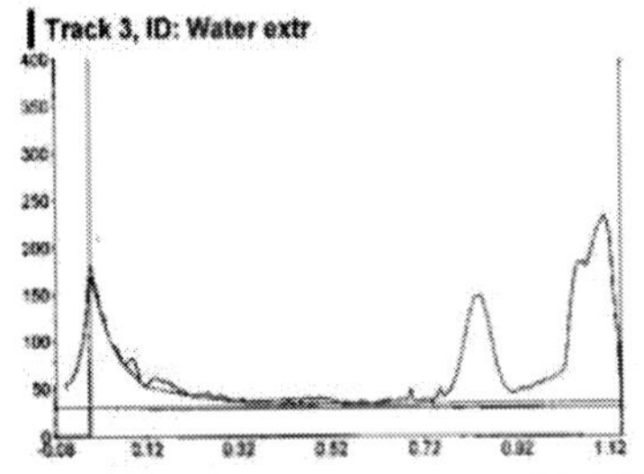

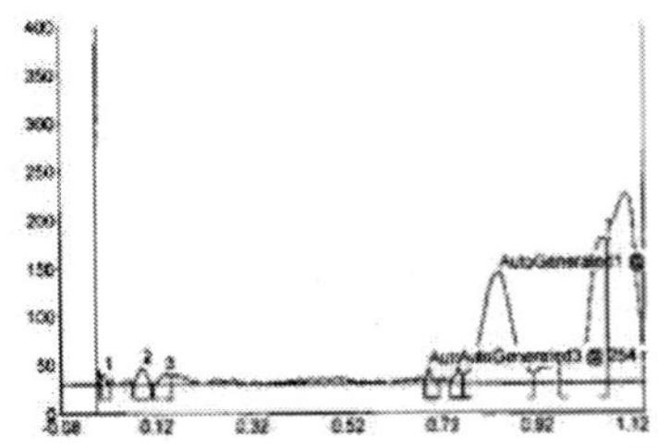

Peak	Start Rf	Start Height	Max Rf	Max Height	Max %	End Rf	End Height	Area	Area %	Assigned Substance
1	0.01	8.4	0.01	10.8	3.21	0.03	1.3	85.8	0.80	unknown*
2	0.08	0.8	0.09	17.5	5.22	0.11	0.2	235.7	2.19	unknown*
3	0.12	0.0	0.14	11.1	3.30	0.16	8.6	172.6	1.61	unknown*
4	0.69	2.9	0.70	15.5	4.60	0.72	3.1	120.5	1.12	AutoGenerated2
5	0.74	2.6	0.76	16.1	4.81	0.77	8.1	156.3	1.45	AutoGenerated3
6	0.77	8.4	0.85	115.1	34.27	0.92	10.3	5433.4	50.55	AutoGenerated1
7	0.97	20.1	1.07	149.8	44.59	1.08	145.8	4543.3	42.27	unknown*

Track 4, ID: Colchicin std-I

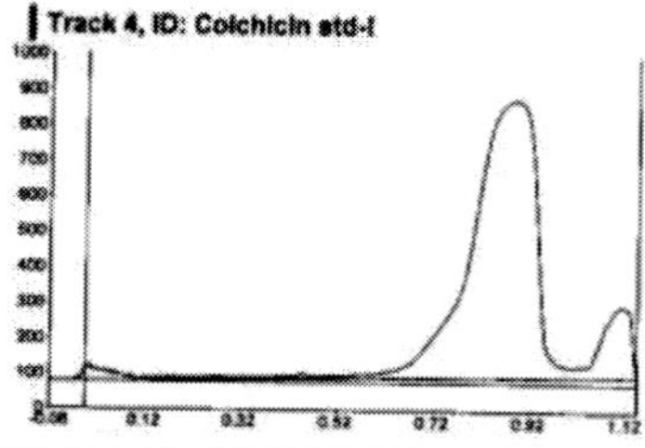

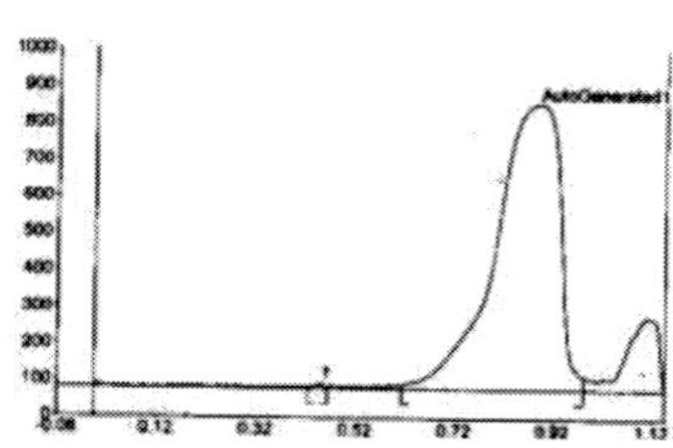

Peak	Start Rf	Start Height	Max Rf	Max Height	Max %	End Rf	End Height	Area	Area %	Assigned Substance
1	0.43	5.2	0.46	15.1	1.91	0.47	4.3	217.6	0.28	unknown*
2	0.62	11.5	0.90	778.6	98.09	0.99	36.3	77541.6	99.72	AutoGenerated1

Track 5, ID: Colchicin std-2

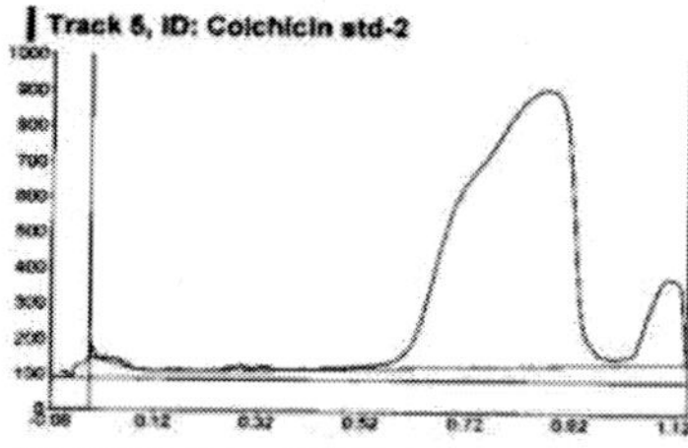

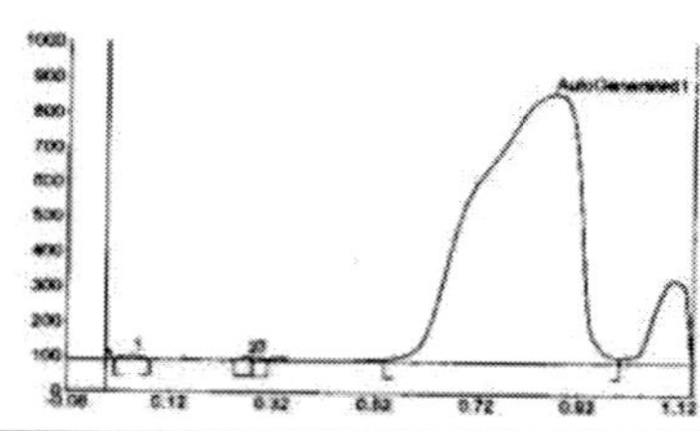

Peak	Start Rf	Start Height	Max Rf	Max Height	Max %	End Rf	End Height	Area	Area %	Assigned Substance
1	0.02	2.5	0.05	14.6	1.79	0.08	0.3	396.8	0.34	unknown*
2	0.25	1.8	0.28	11.6	1.42	0.28	5.3	160.3	0.14	unknown*
3	0.29	5.4	0.29	15.7	1.92	0.32	4.4	184.8	0.16	unknown*
4	0.54	7.4	0.88	774.0	94.87	1.01	16.7	117139.2	99.37	AutoGenerated1

winCATS Planar Chromatography Manager

Toxicology Lab,
IVRI, Izatnagar, Bareilly,
UP, India

Analysis Report

SOP document		
Validated	Design	
Description :		
Analysis	C:\CAMAG\winCATS\Data\I-S.G.Extr.cna	
Created/used by	Supervisor	Tuesday, April 18, 2006 12:07:21 PM
Current user	Supervisor	

Detection - CAMAG TLC Scanner 3

Information

Application position	10.0 mm
Solvent front position	85.0 mm

Instrument	CAMAG TLC Scanner 3 "Scanner3_120716" S/N 120716 (1.14.22)	
Executed by	Supervisor	Tuesday, April 18, 2006 12:06:35 PM
Number of tracks	5	
Position of first track X	10.6 mm	
Distance between tracks	20.0 mm	
Scan start pos. Y	9.1 mm	
Scan end pos. Y	85.0 mm	
Slit dimensions	6.00 x 0.45 mm, Micro	
Optimize optical system	Light	
Scanning speed:	20 mm/s	
Data resolution:	100 µm/step	

Measurement Table

Wavelength	260
Lamp	D2
Measurement Type	Remission
Measurement Mode	Absorption
Optical filter	Second order
Detector mode	Automatic
PM high voltage	290 V

Detector properties

Y-position for 0 adjust	5.0 mm
Track # for 0 adjust	0
Analog Offset	10%
Sensitivity	Automatic (41)

Integration

Properties

Data filtering	Savitsky-Golay 7
Baseline correction	Lowest Slope
Peak threshold min. slope	5
Peak threshold min. height	10 AU
Peak threshold min. area	50
Peak threshold max. height	990 AU
Track start position	11.9 mm
Track end position	85.0 mm
Display scaling	Automatic

winCATS Planar Chromatography Manager

All tracks at Wavelength

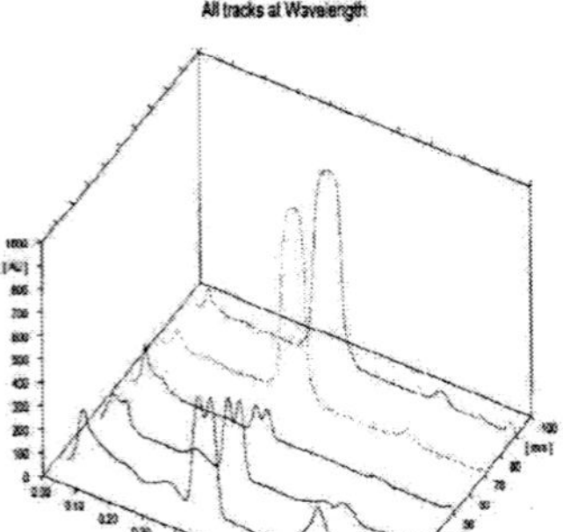

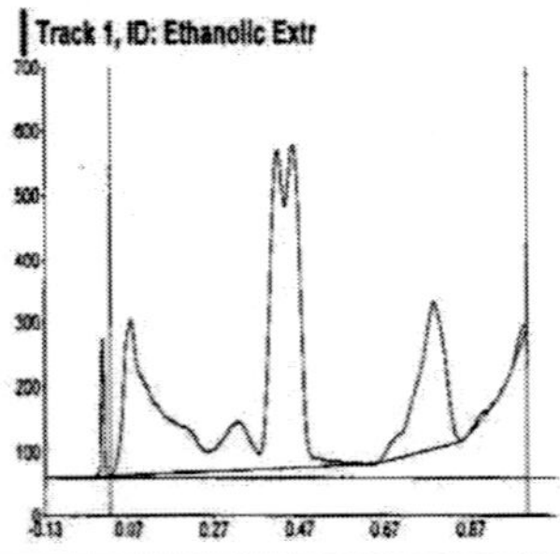

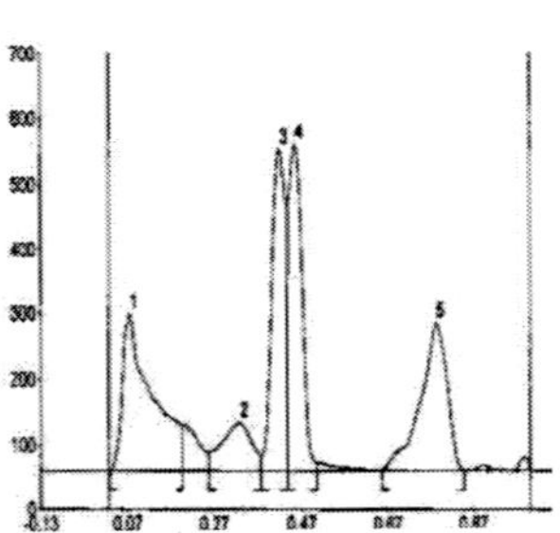

Peak	Start Rf	Start Height	Max Rf	Max Height	Max %	End Rf	End Height	Area	Area %	Assigned Substance
1	0.03	0.4	0.07	239.3	15.60	0.19	70.2	14236.0	24.30	unknown*
2	0.25	29.6	0.33	74.6	4.86	0.37	22.9	4489.1	7.66	unknown*
3	0.37	23.2	0.42	493.5	32.17	0.43	407.3	13524.5	23.09	unknown*
4	0.44	408.9	0.45	501.0	32.67	0.50	12.2	13834.9	23.62	unknown*
5	0.65	1.8	0.78	225.3	14.69	0.85	0.2	12493.8	21.33	unknown*

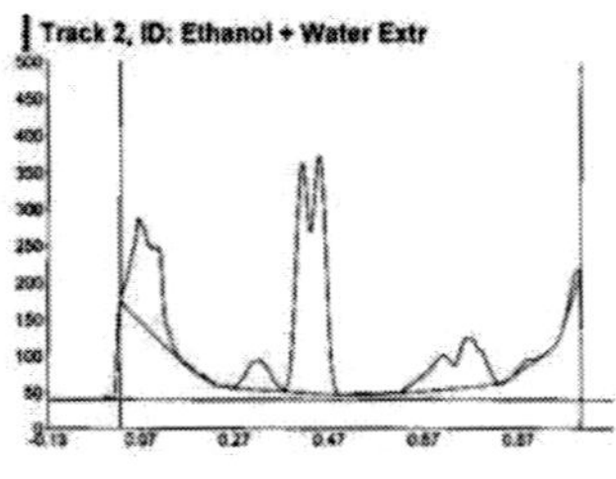

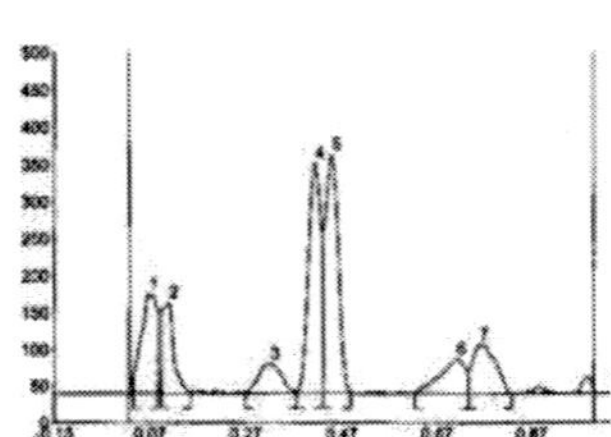

Peak	Start Rf	Start Height	Max Rf	Max Height	Max %	End Rf	End Height	Area	Area %	Assigned Substance
1	0.03	23.9	0.06	136.4	12.95	0.08	114.8	3841.9	13.66	unknown*
2	0.09	114.1	0.11	124.1	11.79	0.15	1.3	2517.9	8.95	unknown*
3	0.27	2.0	0.32	40.9	3.88	0.37	3.3	1713.6	6.16	unknown*
4	0.37	3.4	0.41	312.9	29.71	0.43	220.5	7165.3	25.48	unknown*
5	0.43	221.6	0.45	324.4	30.81	0.49	1.4	7746.3	27.54	unknown*
6	0.62	1.5	0.71	47.6	4.52	0.73	31.2	2201.2	7.83	unknown*
7	0.73	31.5	0.76	66.9	6.35	0.83	0.1	2922.0	10.39	unknown*

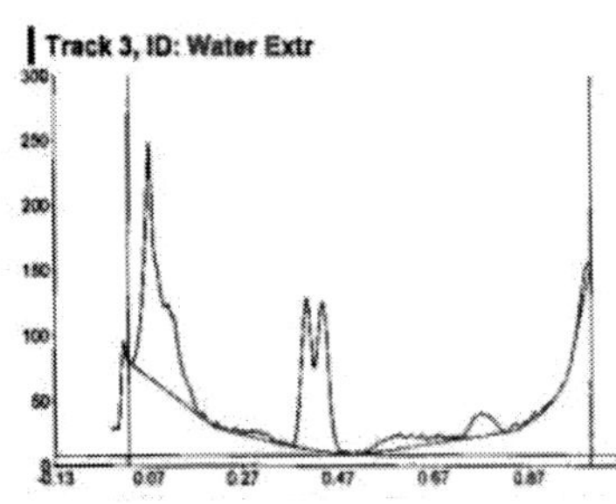

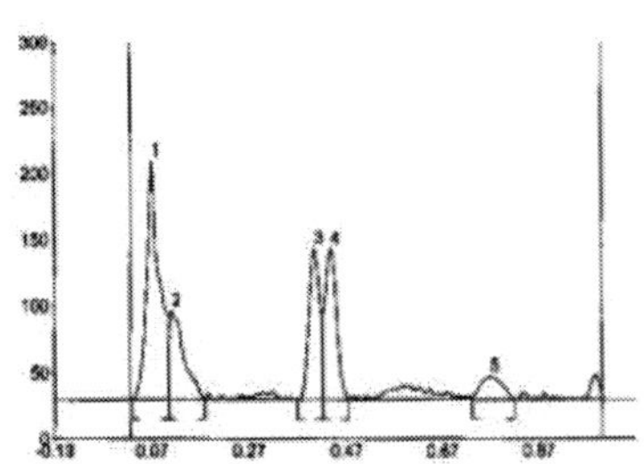

Peak	Start Rf	Start Height	Max Rf	Max Height	Max %	End Rf	End Height	Area	Area %	Assigned Substance
1	0.03	0.1	0.07	179.9	36.58	0.10	62.7	4181.3	37.48	unknown*
2	0.10	63.2	0.11	66.6	13.53	0.18	0.3	1728.6	15.49	unknown*
3	0.37	0.0	0.40	114.1	23.21	0.42	62.6	2216.6	19.87	unknown*
4	0.42	63.2	0.44	113.6	23.10	0.47	1.7	2346.8	21.03	unknown*
5	0.73	1.6	0.77	17.6	3.57	0.82	0.0	684.2	6.13	unknown*

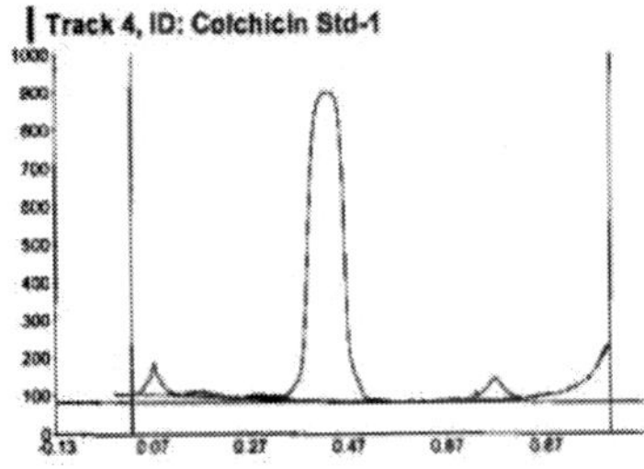

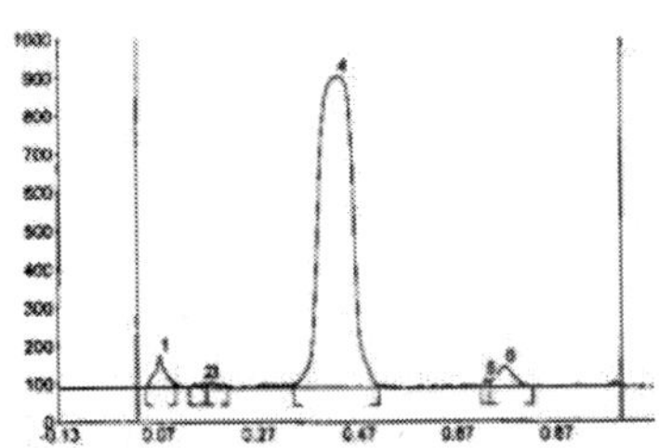

Peak	Start Rf	Start Height	Max Rf	Max Height	Max %	End Rf	End Height	Area	Area %	Assigned Substance
1	0.04	1.6	0.07	83.5	8.35	0.10	9.1	1559.4	3.05	unknown*
2	0.13	1.2	0.16	13.3	1.33	0.16	9.7	200.0	0.39	unknown*
3	0.16	10.0	0.17	12.0	1.20	0.21	3.3	291.4	0.57	unknown*
4	0.34	7.4	0.43	814.2	81.44	0.51	4.7	47344.2	92.46	unknown*
5	0.72	0.6	0.73	22.3	2.23	0.73	10.6	143.0	0.28	unknown*
6	0.73	11.2	0.77	54.6	5.46	0.82	0.1	1665.1	3.25	unknown*

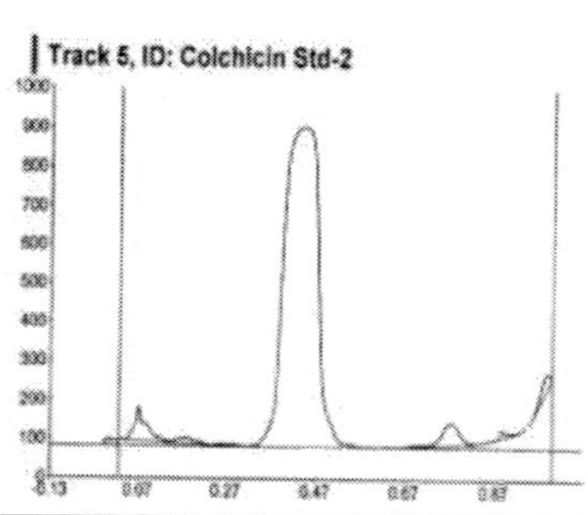

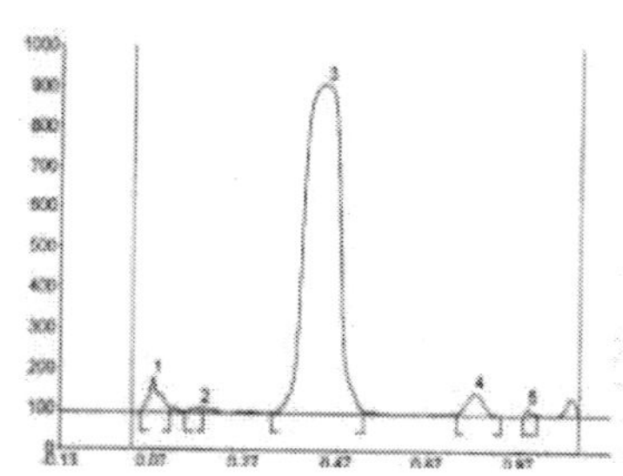

Peak	Start Rf	Start Height	Max Rf	Max Height	Max %	End Rf	End Height	Area	Area %	Assigned Substance
1	0.04	0.7	0.07	86.5	8.68	0.11	12.6	1857.4	3.19	unknown*
2	0.14	2.3	0.17	14.2	1.43	0.18	11.6	262.4	0.45	unknown*
3	0.33	1.9	0.44	818.9	82.14	0.53	9.6	54179.7	92.91	unknown*
4	0.73	3.6	0.77	56.8	5.70	0.83	0.4	1809.6	3.10	unknown*
5	0.88	0.1	0.89	20.6	2.06	0.91	4.9	204.5	0.35	unknown*

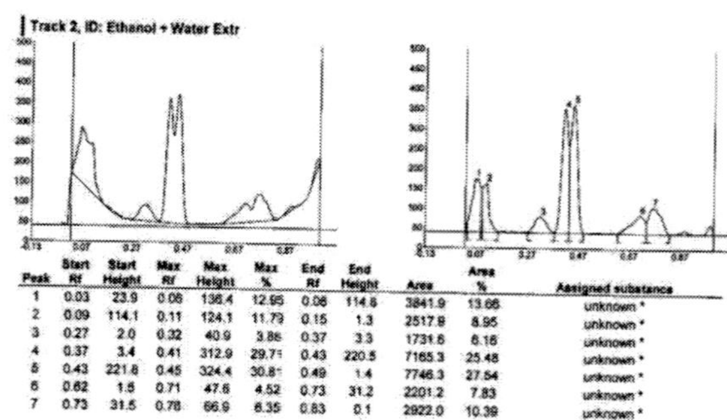

Peak	Start Rf	Start Height	Max Rf	Max Height	Max %	End Rf	End Height	Area	Area %	Assigned substance
1	0.03	23.9	0.08	136.4	12.95	0.08	114.8	3841.9	13.66	unknown *
2	0.09	114.1	0.11	124.1	11.79	0.15	1.3	2517.8	8.95	unknown *
3	0.27	2.0	0.32	40.9	3.88	0.37	3.3	1731.6	6.18	unknown *
4	0.37	3.4	0.41	312.9	29.7[illegible]	0.43	220.5	7165.3	25.48	unknown *
5	0.43	221.8	0.45	324.4	30.8[illegible]	0.49	1.4	7746.3	27.54	unknown *
6	0.62	1.5	0.71	47.8	4.52	0.73	31.2	2201.2	7.83	unknown *
7	0.73	31.5	0.78	66.9	6.35	0.83	0.1	2922.0	10.39	unknown *

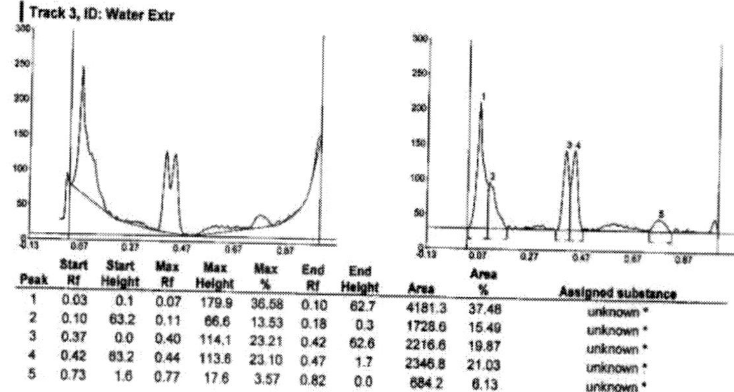

Peak	Start Rf	Start Height	Max Rf	Max Height	Max %	End Rf	End Height	Area	Area %	Assigned substance
1	0.03	0.1	0.07	179.9	36.58	0.10	62.7	4181.3	37.48	unknown *
2	0.10	63.2	0.11	66.6	13.53	0.18	0.3	1728.6	15.49	unknown *
3	0.37	0.0	0.40	114.1	23.21	0.42	62.6	2216.6	19.87	unknown *
4	0.42	63.2	0.44	113.6	23.10	0.47	1.7	2346.8	21.03	unknown *
5	0.73	1.6	0.77	17.6	3.57	0.82	0.0	684.2	6.13	unknown *

Chapter-7

ANTI-INFLAMMATORY ACTIVITY

One of the characteristics of living tissue is its ability to react to injury. The reaction of living tissue to injury which comprises a series of changes of the terminal vascular bed, blood, and connective tissues, which tend to eliminate the injurious agents to repair the damaged tissue, may be called as 'inflammation'. Repair begins during the active phase of inflammation, but reaches completion usually after the injurious influence has been neutralized. Destroyed cells and tissues are repaired thereby. Both inflammation and repair generally serve useful purposes. Without inflammation, bacterial infections would remain un-encountered, wounds would never heal, and injured tissues and organs might be permanently defected. However, inflammation may be potentially harmful. Inflammatory reactions underline the genesis of crippling rheumatoid arthritis, life threatening sensitivity reactions, and some forms of fatal glomerular diseases.

TYPES OF INFLAMMATION

There are two types of inflammation, acute inflammation and chronic inflammation. The classical signs of acute inflammatory reactions are: warmth, redness, pain, swelling and loss of function. The intensity and the localization of the reaction is determined by both severity of the injurious agent and the reactive capacity of the host. Chronic inflammation is also characterized by pain, redness and swelling but it does not subside in a period of days, but may instead have a relentless, damaging course of several weeks, months or years. Mediators of inflammation released from cells are histamine, serotonin, prostaglandin and lysozomal enzymes. Mediators derived from plasma are four major 'cascade' systems the clotting, fibronolytic, kinin and complement systems. Each system has a number of components which include proenzymes, conversion of which to the active enzymes can trigger off the activation of subsequent components in the system, giving a chain or cascade of reaction. Each system is complicated by the presence of inhibitors and accelerators and by positive and negative feedback system. Moreover, some of the activation products of the individual system can interact with the other systems. Each of these systems can make important contributions to the production of an inflammatory condition. (Mukherjee.P.K.,2000)

Various in-vivo and in-vitro models have been proposed as being able to detect anti-inflammatory effect. A few of these methods have been systematically evaluated for their potential usefulness in screening programs and/or have achieved popularity for their ability to select drugs known to exert beneficial effects in rheumatoid diseases. Detailed investigations have been undertaken on several plants for anti-inflammatory activity. The most common screening model has been the prevention of carrageenin induced oedema in rats (Menon et al 1982, Pillai and \santhakumari, 1981).

Usually the paw edema is induced in the hind paw of rats (n=8-12 per group) by sub-plantar injectionof 1% (w/v) lambda carrageenan (Winter et al, 1962). The injected volume is 0.1 ml/rat. The degree of edema is measured immediately before and 3 h after injection of carrageenan by using plethismometer. The difference between the two paw volumes, determined before and after injection of the edema provoking agent indicates the severity of edema (Singh et al 1984, Saxena, 1982).

Carrageenan Induced Rat Paw Edema

1% solution of carrageenan is prepared. 0.1 ml of this solution is to be injected into the right hind paw of the rats (Winter et al, 1962). The test drug/plant extract at varying doses based on the design of the experiment and control vehicle are injected intraperitoneally (i.p.) 30 min. prior to the injection of carrageenan. The paw volume is measured just before and 1. 2, 3, 4, 5h after administration of carrageenan by the volume displacement method (Bhatt et al, 1977), using a plethismometer. For differentiating "counterirritant" activity from "true" anti-inflammatory activity, the test drug/extract is mixed with carrageenan (Mixture I contained specific amount of test drug/extract and 0.1ml of 1% carrageenan; Mixture II contained second dose of extract and 0.1ml of 1% carrageenan) and is injected into the right hind paw of rats (Shanahan, 1968) and the paw volume is measured as before (Bhatt et al, 1977).

Carrageenan induced edema is commonly used as an experimental animal model of acute inflammation and is believed to be biphasic. The first phase is due to release of histamine and serotonin, the second phase is caused by the release of bradykinin, protease, prostaglandin and lysosome (Castro et al, 1968). It has been reported that the second phase of edema is sensitive to most clinically effective anti-inflammatory agents (Smucker et al, 1967). Carrageenan rat paw oedema is a suitable test for evaluating anti-inflammatory drugs which has been frequently used to assess the anti-oedematous effect of natural products. (Delia Loggia ef al, 1986; Alcaraz et al, 1988;Saha et al, 1996).

Apparatus Used for Measuring Volume of Rat Paw (Plethysmometer) Model for Anti-Inflammatory Drug Evaluation A- Prefixed mark on the glass vessel B - Mercury water interface C -U Tube D - Glass Syringe

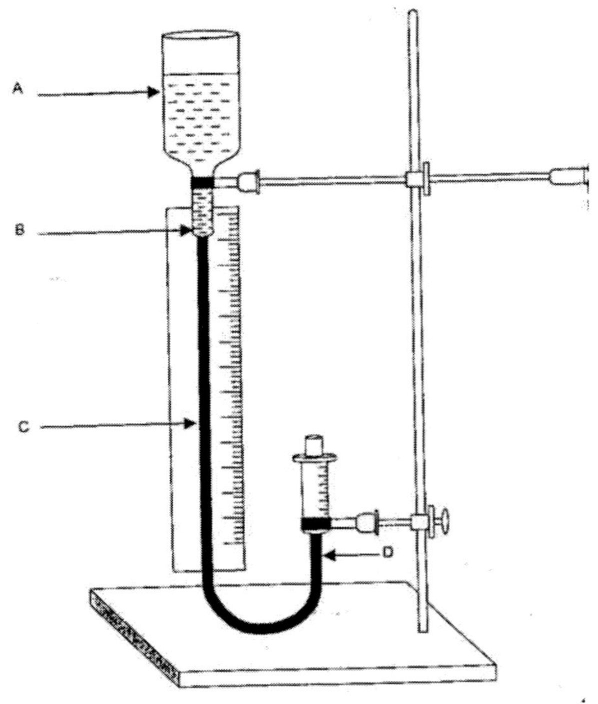

METHODOLOGY

Animal- 25 Male albino rats (200-220gm)

Drug – Carrageenan (1%w/v) solution was prepared and injected 0.1ml of 1%w/v underneath the plantar region.

Standard drug- Indomethacin was selected with a dose of 10mg/kg.

Procedure- The animals were weighed and divided into following groups-

Group-I- Disease control, was treated with 0.1ml of carrageenan (1%solution).

Group-II- The inflammation was induced with 0.1ml of 1%Carrageenan solution and was treated with 10mg/kg of standard drug Indomethacin.

Group-III- The inflammation was induced and treated with 250mg/kg of alcoholic extract of Gloriosa superba Linn.(Tubers)

Group IV- The inflammation was induced with 0.1ml of 1% carrageenan solution and was treated with 250mg/kg of hydroalcoholic extract.

Group-V- The inflammation was induced with 0.1ml of 1% carrageenan solution and was treated with 250mg/kg of aqueous extract.

Before starting the experiment made a mark on the hind paw just beyond tibio-tarsal junction, so that every time the paw was dipped in the mercury column up to the fixed mark to ensure constant volume. Noted the initial paw volume of each rat by mercury displacement method.

After the administration of different drugs to various groups as shown above, 30min. later injected 0.1ml of 1%w/v of carrageenan in the plantar region of the paw of rat. Noted the paw volume of each rat of each group at 0, 30, 60, 90, and 120min. after carrageenan challenge. The difference between two observations gave the amount of edema developed. The percent inhibition of edema for the treated groups was calculated by following formula are compared with the control group.

% Inhibition = 100 X [1 – Vt/Vc]

Where Vt & Vc are the mean changes of paw volume in the treated and control respectively.Here the difference between 0 to 90 min. were taken for the identification of the percent inhibition of edema for the treated groups, with the help of given formula. Results of paw volume changes are given in Table.26.

Table No.26: Effect of test compounds on Carrageenan induce Rat Paw Edema relative increase in Paw volume.

S. No.	Treated Groups	Mean values at different time interval				
		'0'min.	'30'min.	'60'min.	'90'min.	'120'min.
1	Disease Control	0.020± 0.00058	0.066± 0.00040	0.059± 0.00038	0.056± 0.00035	0.035± 0.00032
2	STD	0.024± 0.00057	0.050± 0.00044	0.042± 0.00043	0.030± 0.00044	0.028± 0.00051
3	Extract –I	0.022± 0.00048	0.049± 0.00046	0.041± 0.00043	0.039± 0.00051	0.032± 0.00047
4	Extract-II	0.021± 0.00039	0.050± 0.00044	0.040± 0.00047	0.031± 0.00038	0.028± 0.00058
5	Extract-III	0.022± 0.00055	0.051± 0.00052	0.040± 0.00030	0.030± 0.00028	0.026± 0.00058

Ext.I= Alcoholic Extract, Ext.II= Hydro Alcoholic Extract, Ext. III= Aqueous Extract.

Result- In Carrageenan induced acute model, Indomethacin with a dose of 10 mg/kg served as standard, resulted in 83% inhibition of inflammation.

The alcoholic extract of Gloriosa superba Linn. Tubers, 250mg/kg resulted in 52% inhibition. The hydro alcoholic extract of Gloriosa superba Linn. Tubers, 250mg/kg resulted in 72% inhibition. The aqueous extractn of Gloriosa superba Linn. Tubers, 250mg/kg resulted in 77% inhibition.

Chapter-8

ANTIMICROBIAL ACTIVITY

Antimicrobial activity of plants can be detected by observing the growth response of various' microorganisms to 'those plant tissues or extracts, which are placed in contact with them. Many methods for "detecting such activity are available, but since they are not equally sensitive or even based on the same principle, the results obtained will also be influenced by the method selected and the microorganisms used for the test. It is clear that biological' evaluation in general can be carried out much more efficiently on water-soluble (Janssen et al.,1987;Rios et al.,1988).

In order to detect antimicrobial activity in plant extracts, three conditions must be fulfilled. First, the plant extract must be brought into contact with the cell wall of the microorganisms that have been selected for the test. Second, conditions must be adjusted so that the microorganisms are able to grow when no antimicrobial agents are present. Third, there must be some means of judging the amount of growth, if any, made by the test organism during the period of time chosen for the test (Skinner,1955). The currently available methods for antimicrobial screening fall into three groups viz. diffusion, dilution and bioautographic methods. These methods are influenced by several factors such as extraction method, inocula volume, culture medium composition, pH and incubation temperature. At this point it should be stressed that all available testing methods will only give an idea of the presence or absence of substances with antimicrobial activity in the extract. The potency of the active ingredients can only be determined on pure compounds using a standardized methodology. (mukherjee.P.K.,2000)

Resurgence in the use of herbal medicines worldwide has provided an excellent opportunity to Indian companies to look for therapeutic leads from our ancient system of ayurveda that could be utilized for drug development. Though there are many medicinal plants with anti-microbial properties, only a few have been scientifically evaluated. In maximum cases the crude plant extracts have been taken for anti-microbial screening.

Anti-microbial property of leaf extracts of *Gloriosa superba Linn.* have been reported earlier. Hence, an attempt has been made to investigate the anti-microbial property of Different extracts of gloriosa superba Linn. (Tubers).i.e Ethanolic extract, Ethanol + Water Extract, Water Extract. (Subashini.R.,et.al.,2000)

The present study was carried out to Evaluation of anti-microbial activity of the Different extracts of the *Gloriosa superba Linn.*(Tubbers) against two gram +ve bacteria, two gram-ve bacteria and two fungi. Bacillus subtilis & Bacillus thuringiensis (Gram+ve), Escherichia coli & Pseudomonas aeruginosa (Gram-ve) and Candida albicans & Aspergillus niger (Fungi) were used. (Michael. J.P., et.al.,2000; Aneja.K.R., 1993)

MATERIALS AND METHOD

Agar cup-plate method

1. **Anti-bacterial activity testing**

   The different Extracts of *Gloriosa superba Linn.* (Tubers) were tested for their possible anti-bacterial activity against Bacillus subtilis, Bacillus thuringiensis, Escherichia coli and Pseudomonas aeruginosa. The test was carried out by the agar cup-plate method. Three concentrations (50 mg, 75mg & 100 mg) of the different Extracts were prepared for the antimicrobial screening. Ethanolic extract (F_1) Ethanol+Water extract (F_2) and water extract (A)were dissolved in sterile water. Penicillin (50mg/ml) and Gentamicin (50mg/ml) were used as control for G+ve and G-ve bacteria respectively.

   The anti-bacterial activity was evaluated by employing 24 hrs cultures of above said bacterias using nutrient agar medium. The medium was sterilized by autoclaving at 120°C (PSI). About 30ml of nutrient agar medium inoculated with the respective strains of bacteria (6ml of inoculums to 300ml of nutrient gar medium) was transformed aseptically into each sterile petriplates (10cm diameter). The plates were left at room temperature for solidification. In each plates four wells of 6mm diameter were made using sterile borer. Accurately 0.2ml of the test and standard solutions were transferred to cups aseptically and labeled accordingly. The plates were then maintained at room temperature for 2hrs to allow the diffusion of the solution into the medium. The petriplates used for anti-bacterial screening were incubated at 37±1°C for 24hrs. The diameter of zone of inhibition surrounding each of the wells was recorded. (Mensah.A.Y.,et.al.,2000; Mensah.A.Y.,et.al.,2001)

2. **Anti-fungal Activity test**

All the Extracts were tested for their possible anti-fungal activity against Candida albicans and Aspergillus niger. The test was carried out by the agar cup-plate method. Three concentrations (50 mg, 75mg & 100 mg) of the different Extracts were prepared for the antifungal screening. Ethanolic extract (F_1) Ethanol+Water extract (F_2) and Water extract (A)were dissolved in sterile water.Ketoconazole (50mg/ml) was used as control for both the fungus. The anti-fungal activity was evaluated by employing 48hrs cultures of above said fungus using nutrient agar medium. The petriplates were incubated at 37±1°C for 48 hrs. The diameter of zone of inhibition surrounding each of the wells was recorded. (Carter.S.J., 2000)

RESULT

The Ethanolic, Ethanol+Water and water extracts of *Gloriosa superba Linn.* (Tubers) Showed good antibacterial activity and anti fungal activity as shown in the Table.27.

ANTIMICROBIAL SCREENING

Agar Cup-plate method

Table No. 27: Zone of inhibition of various microorganisms against various Extracts of the *Gloriosa superba Linn.* (Tubers)

S. No.	Organisms	Extract-I (F1)			Extract –II (F2)			Extract-III (A)			P	G	K
		50µg	75µg	100µg	50µg	75µg	100µg	50µg	75µg	100µg	50µg	50µg	50µg
1	E.coli	12	10	14	12	12	14	08	13	15	-	22	-
2	P.aeruginosa	14	16	16	10	10	10	08	13	14	-	23	-
3	B.subtilis	18	18	23	14	16	19	20	24	24	25	-	-
4	B.thuringiensis	21	21	23	14	16	18	20	22	26	32	-	-
5	A.niger	R	R	R	11	11	11	08	11	11	-	-	18
6	C.albicans	R	R	R	R	R	R	R	R	08	-	-	08

Key:-

a. Measurement unit were millimeter
b. Extract-I (F1) =Ethanolic Extract
c. Extract-II (F2) = Ethanol + Water Extract
d. Extract-III (A) = Water Extract
e. P= Penicillin
f. G= Gentamicin
g. K= Ketoconazole
h. R= Resistant

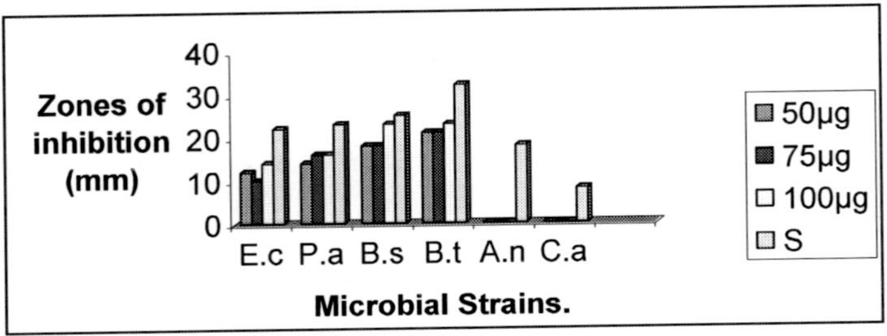

Fig 3: Zone of inhibition of various microorganism against Extract-I

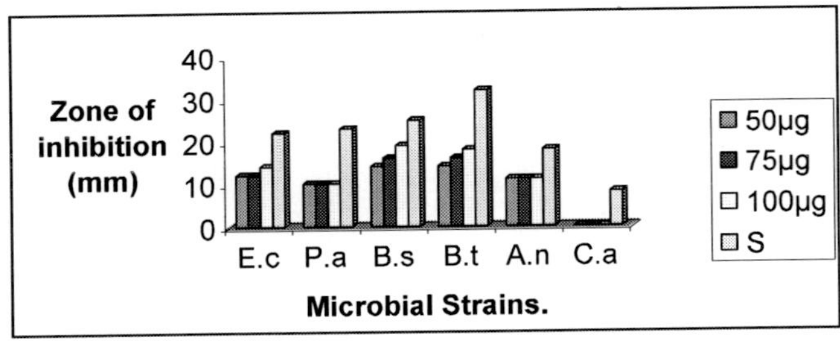

Fig 4: Zone of inhibition of various microorganism against Extract-II

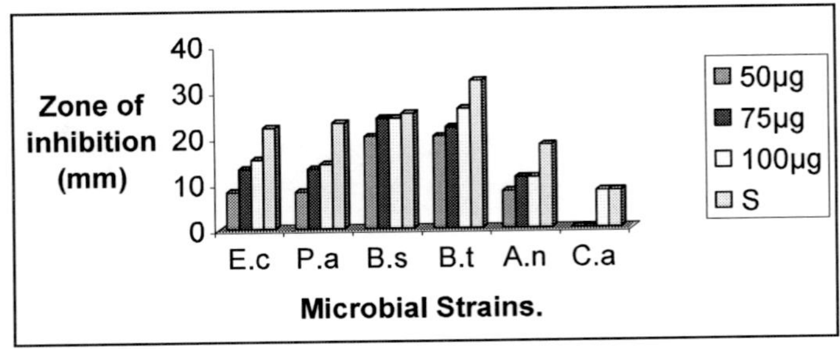

Fig 5: Zone of inhibition of various microorganism against Extract-III

Chapter-9

SUMMARY & CONCLUSION

The investigation related to *Gloriosa superba Linn.* is proposed that the plant is tall herbaceous climber. This is found in throughout tropical India.

The plant tubers are very long, solid, white yellowish in colour and having characteristics odour and it is used as abortifacient, anti-inflammatory, anti-microbial and in the treatment of rheumatism, skin diseases, leprosy, white discharge.

The present investigation under taken with a view of explore the standardization, phytochemical screening, and bring force pharmacological activity of plant tubers.

The tubers of *Gloriosa superba Linn.* Were collected in month of December from Distt. Jhansi U.P. The tubers were authenticated by morphological and microscopic characters along with powder analysis.

The extractive values were found by hot and cold extraction methods. The ash value, loss on drying, Swelling index, foaming index, microbial contamination are other parameter of standardization. The volatile oil were absent in the Tubers.

The coarse powder of Tubers were extracted by Alcohol (90%), Hydro-alcohol (60 : 40 - Alcohol : water) and Aqueous Solvents. The alcohol and Hydroalcohol extract give more constituents and more effective.

Generally all extracts contain Alkaloids, Carbohydrates, Glycosides, amino acids, organic acids, steroid & saponine etc.

All the extract was investigated by TLC. The best resolution of alcoholic and hydro alcoholic extracts were found when Ethylacetate: Glacial acetic acid: formic acid: water: (100:10:10:27) solvent system and silica gel G as absorbent used. In case of aqueous extract the solvent system was ethyl acetate : methanol : water (100:13.5:10) used. These solvent system resolved the extract in 4-5 spots.

After the TLC all extract were analyzed by HPTLC and get fine resolution of all extract.

All extract were exhibited good antimicrobial activity and antifungal activity. The antimicrobial activity was performed by Agar cup-plate method. The standard antimicrobial drug, Penicillin taken in 50 µg, Gentamicin taken 50µg. The standard antifungal drug ketoconazole 50µg was taken. The dose of extracts were taken 50µg, 75µg,100µg.

Good anti-inflammatory action was showed by all extracts of *Gloriosa superba Linn. Tubers.* The doses of extracts were taken 250mg/kg and standard Indomethacin was given 10 mg/kg orally. And all extract of *Gloriosa superba Linn. Tubers.* show good anti-inflammatory activity.

Chapter-10

BIBLIOGRAPHY

1. Alacanz, M.J.; Jimenez, M.J.; (1988) Flavonoids as anti inflammatory agent, *Fitoterapia,* 59, 75-38.
2. Amal,J.A.;Bhavani Sanker,K.;Gloriosa superba.-A Talisman for Leprosy and Cancer, National Conferece on recent Trendsa in Spices & Medicinal plant Reseach,Calcutta,WB,India,A-76,2-4 April 1998.
3. Antony, R; Torkelson.; The cross name Index to medicinal plants V. 3, 1996.
4. Aneja, K.R.; Experimental in microbiology, plant pathology and tissue culture, P.36-44, 1993.
5. Arambewela, L.S.R.; Kumudini, M.A.N.; Ranatunga, J.; *Journal of the National Science Concil of Sri Lanka*, V. 19 (2): P. 177-180, 1991.
6. Bhatt, K.R.; Mehata, R.K.; Srivastava, P.N.;(1977) A simple method for recording anti inflammatory effect in rat paw oedema, *Indian J. Physiol. Pharm*, 21, 399-400.
7. Caroline, K; Hatton.; Pharmacognosy, Phytochemistry of Medicinal plant., 2nd edi. P. 952-955. (1999)
8. Carter, S.J.; Tutorial Pharmacy, 6th edi. 2000.
9. Castro, J.; Sasame, H.; et. al., (1968) Diverse effect of SKF 52 and antioxidant on CCl4 induced changes... metabolism, Life Sci, 7, 129-136.
10. Chandravadana,M.V.;Sebastian,E.;Nidiry,J.; Lella,N.K.; Parvatha Reddy, P.;Khan, R.M.; Rao, M.S; Nematicidal activity of some plant extracts., *Indian Journal Of Nematology*,V.26(2):P.148-151,1996.
11. Chaudhari,P.K.; Nonalkaloidal constituents of the seeds of Gloriosa superba.,*Indian Journal of Chemistry*,V.37 B(1):P.98-99.1998
12. Chaudhuri, P.K.; Colchicine from Gloriosa superba Linn. A substitute of Colchicum autumnale Linn., *Indian drug.* V.30(10):P.529-530,1993.
13. Chaudhuri, P.K.;Thakur, R.S.; 1,2-Di demethyl Colchicine: A new alkaloid from Gloriosa superba, *Journal Of Natural Products*,V.56(7);P.1174-1176, 1993.

14. Chauhan,S.K.;Singh,A.P.;Agrawal,S.; Development of HPTLC methods for the estimation of colchicines in different parts of Gloriosa superba, *In dianDrugs*,V.35(5):P.266-268,1998.
15. Chopra, R.N.;Nayar,S.L;and Chopra,I.C.; *Glossary of Indian Medicinal Plants* CSIR New Delhi,1956,P.125-126.
16. Clewer, Green and Tutin reported the isolation of colchicine and two other alkaloids from the dried tubers of Gloriosa superba, collected from ceyclon *J.Sci. Industrial Res.* Vol., 11B, 1952, 446-447.
17. De- Eknamkul,W.;Kitcharoen,N.; Colchicine content in the seeds and various parts of Thi Gloriosa superba., *Phytomedicine*,V.3(suppl.1); P.192,1996/97.
18. Della-Loggia, A; Tubero, A., et. al., (1986) the role of flavonoils in the anti inflammatory activity of chamomilla recutita, *Clin. Biol. Res*, 213, 481-488.
19. Duke.;James, A;*Hand book of Medicinal Herbs*.P.213-214.(1929).
20. Devagiri, G.M.; Patil, S.K.; Dabgar, V.M.; Shivanna, H.; Influence of hormone on rooting of Gloriosa superba stem cuttings, *Indian Drugs*, V.36(6),P.479-480,1999.
21. Egon stahl.; TLC- A laboratory hand book Iind Edi.; P.421, 2005.
22. Farooqi,A.A.;Gowda,H.R.;Hegde,L;*Journal Of Medicinal and Aromatic Plant Sciences*,V.21(2);P.316-319,1999.
23. Farooqui, A.A; Kumara swamy, B.K; Bajappa, K.N; Pusalkar, V.R; Gupta, R; *Indian Horticulture*, V. 37(4): P. 26-29, 1993.
24. Gupta,K.R.;Kotagale, N.R.;Saoji, A.N.; Waikar,S.B.; Wadodkar, S.G., Hepatoprotective activity of *Gloriosa superba Linn.*, National Convention on Current Trends in Herbal Drugs &Annual Conference of India Society of Pharmacognosy; Herb; The Natural Altarnative, Gandhinagar, Gujarat, India, P.P-10, January 17-18,2003.
25. Henry, G; Greenish; *Materia Medica*; Edi-3. P.186-188. 1999.
26. *Indian Pharmacopoeia.*; V. I (A-0) (1996)
27. Iyengar, M.A; Nayak, S.G.K., 8th Edition (2001).
28. Iyengar, M.A.; Pharmacognosy of powdered crude Drugs.(2001)
29. Jadhav, S.Y.; and Hegde, B.A,; *Indian Journal of Experimental Biology* V. 39. P. 943-946,2001
30. Jain, A.K; Patole, S.N; *Ethnobotany*, V. 13 (1 & 2): P. 96-100, 2001.
31. Janssen, A.M; Scheffer, J.J.C; Baerheim, S.A; (1987) *Planta Medica*, 53, 395-398.
32. Janssen, A.M; Scheffer, J.J.C; Baerheim, S.A; (1986) Progress in essential oil Research, L.J. Brunke ed, Walter D, Gruyter, Berlin, 419.
33. Kapoor, L.D; Hand book of Ayurvedic medicinal plant.
34. Kay, L.A.;The Microscopical study of drug., 1938.
35. Khandelwal, K.R; practical Pharmacognosy August, p.149-156, 2002.

36. Khory,R.N.,et.al.;*Materia Medica of India*.P.614-615.
37. Kokate, C.K.; Purohit, A.P.; Gokhale, S.B; *Text book of Pharmacognosy*, P-504-506. 2001.
38. Kumaraswamy, B.K; Bhojappa, K.M; and Faraoqi, A.A; *Indian Journal of Forestry V.* 17(3): P-249-251, 1994.
39. Lever, M; Vander Bargh Da, et al; (1979) *Planta medica*, 36, 311-321.
40. Linton, A.H., (1983) Antibiotics: Assessment of Anti microbial Activity and Resistance, AD Russell and LB Quesnel ed, Academic press, London, 19-30.
41. Menon, P.S; Gangabai, G; Swarnalakshmi, T; (1982) chemical and pharmacological studies on peltophorum pterocarpum, *Indian Drug,* 19, 345-347.
42. Mensah, A.Y., et. al.; (2000*) J. Natural product* 63, 1210-1213.
43. Mensah, A.Y., et. al.; (2001*) J. Ethano Pharmacology* 77, 219-226.
44. Michael, J. Pelczar.; J.R; Chan, E.C.S. Krieg, Noel. R; (2000) 5th edi.
45. Mitscher, L.A.; Leu, R.P., et. al.; (1972) Lloydia, 35, 157-166.
46. Mukherjee,Pulok.K;*Quality Control of Herbal Drugs*. P-735-737.
47. Nidiry, E.S.I.;Khan, R.M.; Reddy,P.P.; Invitro nematicidal activity of Gloriosa superba Seed extract against Meloidogyne incognita, *Nematologia Mediteranea*,V.21(2); P.127-128,1993.
48. Onawunmi, G.O.; Yasak, W.; Ogunlana, E.O; (1984) *J. Ethnopharmacol*, 12, 279-186.
49. Parmar, N.S.; Ghosh, M.N.; (1978) Anti inflammatory activity of gossipin bioflavonoid isolated from Hibiscus vitifolius, *Indian J. Pharmacol,* 10, 277-293.*Planta medica* 1994 Feb; 60 (i): 77-83.
50. Poulev,A.;Deus-Neuman,B.;Bombadelli,E.;Zenk,M.H.;Immunoassays for the quantitative determination of colchicines., *Planta, Medica* V.60(1); P.77-83, 1994.
51. Puspangadan, U.L.F; Nyman, V.;George *Glimpses of Indian Ethno Pharmacology*, 562-595, 1995.
52. Raina, R., Sharma, S., Gupta, I.; *M J. of Medicinal and Aromatic plant sciences*, V. 22. P. 85-86, 2000.
53. Rajan,Vinay,Jain,S.k.; *Fourth International Cong.Ethnobiol.,NBRI Lucknow,* P.286, 17-21 Nov.1994.
54. Rios, J.J.; Recio, M.C.; Villard, A.; (1988) *J. Ethnopharmacology*, 23, 127-148.
55. Saha, K.; Mukherjee, P.K.; Das, J.; Mandal, S.C.; Pal, M.; Saha, B.P; (1996) Anti inflammatory evaluation of Leucas lavandulaefolia Rees extract, *Natural Product sciences*, 2(2), 119-122.
56. Saily,A.;Sahu,;Gupta,B.;Sondhi,S.M.; Analysis for mineral elements of medicinal plant used for the treatment of Asthma, Syphilis, Diarrhoea, Skin diseases and Rheumatism *Hamdard Medicus*, V.34(4);P.18-22,1994.

57. Samarajeewa, P.K.; Dassanayake, M.D.; Jayawardena, D.G.; Clonal propagation of *Gloriosa superba Linn.* Indian Journal of Experimental Biology, V.31(8):P.719-720, 1993.
58. Saravanan, S.; Buvaneswaran, C.; *Advances in plant sciences*, V. 16(1): P. 23-28, 2003.
59. Saxena, R.C.; Nath, R.; (1982) Effect of calophylloide a non-steroidal anti-inflammatory agent on capillary permeability, *Planta medica*, 44, 246-248.
60. Shanahan, R.W.; (1968) Local activity of anti inflammatory...By carrageenin, *Arch. Inter. Pharma. Terap*, 175, 189-192.
61. Sharma, A.K.; Gupta, B.K.; Suri, J.L.; Gupta, G.K.; and Atal, C.K.; *Indian Drug*, 24 (3) P. 129-131, 1986.
62. Singh, G.B.; Kaur, S.; (1984) Anti inflammatory activity of Euphorbia acaulis, *J. Ethnopharmacol*, 10, 225-233.
63. Siva Kumar,G.; Krishnamurthy, K.V.; Rajendran,T.D.; Embryoidogenesis and plant regeneration from leaf tissue of Gloriosa superba. *Planta Medica*, V.69(5), P.479-481, 2003.
64. Skinner, F.A.; (1955) Moderne methoden der pflanzennalyse, K. Peach, MV tracey ed, Vol 3, 626-725, Springer verlag, Germany.
65. Smucker, E.; Arrhenous, E.; Hiltin, T.; (1967) Alteration in microsomal electron transport induced by liver injury, *Biochem, J.*, 103, 55-64.
66. Somani, V.J.; John, C.K.;Thengane, R.J.; *Indian Journal of Experimental Biology* V.27. P.578-579. 1989.
67. Stahl, E.; Thin layer chromatography, 1965.
68. Subashini, R.; Manimara, S.;Ruckmani, K.; Antimicrobial activity of leaf extraction of *Gloriosa superba Linn.*, Proceedings of International Congress on " Ayurveda 2000" Chennai,TN,India, P.216, January 28-30, 2000.
69. Suganthi, C.P.; Vijayalakshmi, P.; Reddy, V.R.; Effect of rhizome extract of *Gloriosa superba Linn.* On Allium., Advances in plant sciences,V. 6(1):P.54-59, 1993.
70. Sukh, Dev.; Ethnobotanical survey of traditional plants, *current sscience*, 73, 909-928,1997.
71. Swarmapriya, R.; Doraipandian, A.; Arumugam, T.; Radha, N.S.; *South Indian Horticulture*, V. 43 (1 & 2): P. 40-41, 1995.
72. Swingle, K.T.; (1974) Evaluation for anti inflammatory activity, Anti inflammatory Agents-Chemistry and Pharmacology, R.A. scherre, M.W. white house ed, Academic press, NY, 34-122.
73. Thakur, R.S.; potesilova, H.; and Santavy, F.; *Planta medica V.* 28, p-201-8 (1975).
74. Vijaya Valli, B.; Mathew, P.M.; *The nucleus* V. 35 (1) p. 55-58, 1992.
75. Vasishta, P.C.; Text book of plant Anatomy P.387-389, 1993.

76. Wagner, H.; Bladt, S.; Plant Drug Analysis, 2nd ed. P-40.2002.
77. Washington, J.A; (1988) Diagn. Microbiol Dis., 9, 135-138.
78. Wealth of India,First supplement series (Raw materials) (D-I) v.3 P.178-180, 2002.
79. *World Health Organization,* Geneva.,2002.
80. Winter, C.A.; Porter. C.C; (1975) Effect of alteration inside chain upon anti inflammatory and liver glycogen activity of hydrocortisone ester, *J. Am. Pharm. Ass*, 46, 515-519.
81. Winter, C.A.; Risley, E.A.; Nuss, G.W.; (1962) Carrageenan induced oedema in hind paw as an assay for anti inflammatory drugs, Proc. *Soc. Exp. Biol. Med*, 111, 544-547.
82. WWW. Ethnobotany. Com. Accessing date 4th June, 2005.
83. Yelne, M.B.;Sharma, P.C.; In vitro propagation of medicinal plants: advantages, disadvantages and constraints. South east asian seminar on herbs and herbal medicines, Patna, P.134, 16-19 Jan 1999.